Are You Kidney(ing) Me

*My Personal Experience
with Kidney Disease*

EL JAI MACOY

Copyright © 2024 El Jai Macoy
All rights reserved
First Edition

Fulton Books
Meadville, PA

Published by Fulton Books 2024

ISBN 979-8-89427-017-3 (paperback)
ISBN 979-8-89427-018-0 (digital)

Printed in the United States of America

This book is dedicated to all the deceased and living kidney donors and those individuals still living with end-stage renal disease (ERSD). To the doctors, nurses, technicians, volunteers, and supporters who labor so diligently in this field of care, God bless you all.

And to my children, Daddy loves you.

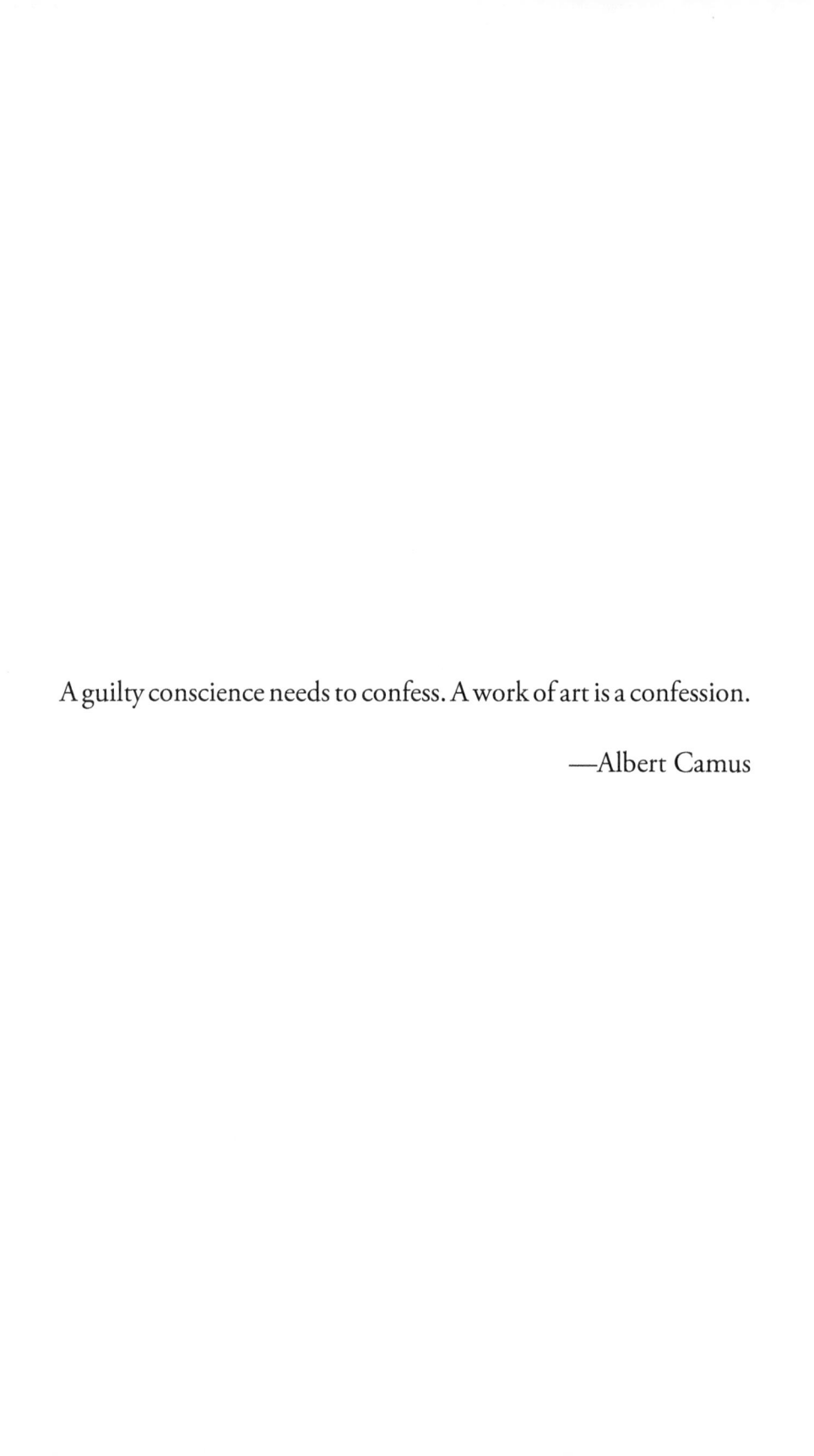

A guilty conscience needs to confess. A work of art is a confession.

—Albert Camus

CONTENTS

Preface vii
Chapter 1:   Prognosis: I'll be all Right 1
Chapter 2:   Diagnosis: Who Me? 7
Chapter 3:   Reality Check/Nephro Please! 17
Chapter 4:   Information Overload 27
Chapter 5:   Treatment: Win the Morning, Win the Day.... 39
Chapter 6:   Upside to the Downside 48
Chapter 7:   Getting Testy 56
Chapter 8:   Wait and Believe 64
Chapter 9:   I Struck a Match 69
Chapter 10: Transplantation 77
Chapter 11: Another Beginning 85
Chapter 12: Better to Give than to Receive 94
Quick Kidney Disease Facts and Stats 98

PREFACE

Why I Decided to Write This Book

Imagine waking up one day and finding out that your kidneys are failing, that you have a life-threatening condition that requires constant treatment, that you have to make drastic changes in your lifestyle, and that you have to face the possibility of losing your life. That's what happened to me when I was fifty-eight years old. This book is not a medical guide or a self-help book. It is a personal story of how I learned that I had kidney failure. I want to share my experience with you, not to scare you or make you feel sorry for me but to encourage you and give you hope.

You see, I was one of those people who thought they were healthy as a horse, and I had nothing to worry about. I ate well, exercised regularly, drank moderately, and avoided smoking. I had no symptoms, no pain, and no problems. Until one day, I was told the shocking news: I had chronic kidney disease, and I needed dialysis or a transplant to survive.

I was stunned. How could this happen to me? What did I do wrong? What could I have done differently? These questions haunted me for a long time, until I realized that there was no point in dwelling on the past. What mattered was the present and the future. How could I cope with this new reality? How could I make the best of it? How could I help others who were going through the same thing?

In this book, you will read about how I discovered my condition, what symptoms I had, how I prepare and cope with the treatments, what to expect from them, and how I found support and inspiration from others to keep the faith and to never give up hope.

So if you are going through the same health issue or know someone who is, you are not alone. There are many people who understand what you are feeling and who can support you. You can also help others by sharing your story, raising awareness, donating money or organs, volunteering for organizations, or joining support groups. You can make a positive impact in the world by helping others who are facing kidney failure or other health challenges.

For those of you who are still healthy, you have a chance to prevent or delay kidney failure by making some changes in your lifestyle. I made some mistakes that I regret, and I hope you can learn from them and avoid them. This is one of the main messages I want to convey in this book.

One of the most important parts of my story is the treatment options offered to me for my kidney failure—conservative care, dialysis, and transplantation. I will discuss the pros and cons of each and how they affected my physical and mental health. The treatments are not easy—they require a lot of time, money, and commitment. They also have side effects and risks. Sometimes I felt tired, depressed, angry, or hopeless. Sometimes I wanted to give up. But I also learned to appreciate the benefits of the treatments. They help me survive, improve my quality of life, and give me a chance for a better future. They also taught me some valuable lessons about gratitude, resilience, and faith.

If you are a kidney patient or a caregiver or a friend or a curious bystander, I invite you to read this book. You will find stories that will make you cry, stories that will make you smile, and stories that will make you think. You will also find tips and advice on how to deal with kidney disease, how to stay positive, how to enjoy life, and how to support others.

I hope that by reading this book, you will feel inspired, encouraged, and entertained, and most of all, I hope that you will realize that you are not alone in this journey. We are all in this together, and we can make it through.

One more thing: I want to show you that life is not over when you have kidney disease. It's just different.

Contributors to this book

Written by one, inspired by many.

CHAPTER 1

Prognosis
I'll Be All Right

Let me start by saying I am a patient; I am not a doctor. Like most things in life, experiences vary from person to person; this is *my* experience.

It was the third day of the new year and the day before my return to the United States after a seven-day vacation on a beautiful Caribbean island, an island where the sea and sky appear to merge to paint a masterful blue canvas with alabaster clouds strategically scattered throughout the sky—the clouds supplying timely reprieves from the blazing hot, radiant sun. It was a week of peaceful morning walks on the beach accompanied only by seagulls and the endless ebb and flow of the waves—the type of morning where the moon barely beats the sun home. The evenings were equally majestic with moonlit skies, an occasional palatial-like yacht on the distant horizon, and an array of stars that would make one forget that Hollywood ever existed.

A negative COVID-19 test was required before reentering the country. That morning, I woke up, and my thumb, index, and middle finger on my left hand were numb, as well as the left side of my mouth. I thought I had slept too long on that side and believed once I moved around, the feeling in my digits and lips would return to normal, but as I stood and walked around, I didn't feel as surefooted as I usually felt.

I remember calling my daughter (who is a physician by the way) later that afternoon (incidentally one of the most expensive calls I've ever made—word to the wise, think twice before making an international phone call), and her advice was to get medical help as I may have had a stroke. I said, "No, I'll be all right, and besides, I'll be back home tomorrow, and I don't want to go to a hospital in a foreign country."

The next day, the symptoms remained, and I remember feeling so disoriented standing in the customs line, which seemed to take forever but was closer to ninety minutes (about an hour and a half). When I returned to the States, I still didn't feel quite right and decided to make an appointment with my new primary care physician (PCP).

I was so confident (substitute arrogant or ignorant) about my health that I had retired a year and a half earlier at the age of fifty-six with no medical insurance, believing that I could maintain my health until I became eligible for Medicare in nine years. I reasoned that any incidental health-care needs that may arise could be taken care of out of pocket. Well, fortunately for me, in March of the year following my early retirement, the state of Maryland offered open enrollment for health insurance to all residents due to the coronavirus disease of 2019, better known as COVID-19, so I was without health insurance for only eight months.

The appointment with my new PCP was scheduled for January 21st, and I informed the PCP of my holiday ordeal. I underwent a standard physical including blood work, and he referred me to a neurologist (brain, spinal cord, and nervous system doctor) to verify if I indeed had a stroke. He also recommended that I schedule an appointment with a nephrologist (a kidney doctor). What does he see in my blood work? Why is he referring me to a nephrologist? I came here to find out why my hand and face are numb.

Anyway, I was able to meet with the neurologist one week later on the 28th. I said to myself, "I like my new PCP. This guy doesn't mess around." The neurologist's notes (abbreviated here) were as follows:

> Progress Notes by Dr. D at 1/28/2022 8:15 AM
> I was called by Dr. M who states this is a new patient for him and the patient states on 1/3/22 he had acute onset L face, L hand numbness and also dropping things from L hand. Patients with stroke risk of HTN (hypertension), HLD (hyperlipidemia/ high cholesterol), and DM (diabetes mellitus). His symptoms resolved. The patient is on ASA 81mg daily and Dr. M is restarting his statin and ordered him a BP cuff to make sure stable at home. FLP (full lipid panel) and HGBA1c are also on order.
>
> **History of Present Illness:**
> The patient is a 58 y.o. male who on 1/3/22 woke up with numbness on the L side of his face and L hand. The patient still has the sensation. He felt that first week he did not feel "sure-footed." So he followed up with PCP last week and recommended a visit with Neurology.
> He was hospitalized at JH in Oct 2020 with pseudogout in the RH and infection. He was admitted for 4 days.
> He had seen an endocrinologist over the summer who told him he was fine and did not

need medication. He has kidney issues, so they were hesitant to start blood sugar medication.

His blood pressure at home is 140s/90s most of the time. Sometimes it goes up to 160s.

Stroke risk factors:
Hypertension: present
Hyperlipidemia: present
Diabetes: present elevated HGBA1c
Smoking: present remote quit 20 years ago
Family history: present

Past Medical History:
Diagnosis Date
- Chronic kidney disease 03/01/2020
- Diabetes mellitus 10/10/2020 Managing via diet
- Hyperlipidemia 05/20/2021
- Hypertension 10/10/2020
- Stroke 01/03/2022

Not sure about this—numbness on the left side of the face

Assessment:
Patient is a 58 y.o. male with stroke like symptoms for the last month with numbness on the L face and L hand. Today we discussed causes of stroke and signs and symptoms of stroke. You have multiple stroke risks that are currently not under control including your blood pressure and elevated blood sugars. Fortunately, you no longer use tobacco but

do have a family history of stroke. Your exam does have findings of possible small vessel stroke as the numbness does not map out to a specific nerve group and it includes your face and hand.

EKG and echocardiogram were done in October and did not show cause for stroke. Further work-up is needed at this time.

Plan: We discussed the following recommendations:
1. Agree with MRI brain which is scheduled for tonight. Please make sure this office gets a copy of the report
2. Carotid ultrasound
3. Continue aspirin 81mg a day and your statin
4. Keep a log of your blood pressures and work with PCP to get the numbers near normal
5. Call PCP if you cannot get in with your endocrinologist to work on blood sugar control options or call the endocrinologist and let them know we are worried you had a small stroke and see if they can get you in sooner
6. Signs and symptoms of stroke reviewed
7. Please go to ED (emergency dept) if you have new stroke symptoms in the future

Follow up: 3 months
DR. D, MD FAHA GBMC Center for Neurology
1/28/2022 at 8:33 AM
Total time on date of service 55 minutes.

After reviewing my labs as well as the neurologist's assessment, my PCP reiterated his desire for me to schedule a follow-up appointment with the nephrologist, again with the doggone nephrologist. What is going on with my kidneys?

He had concerns with my blood glucose, blood pressure, and creatinine levels, so in an abundance of caution, the blood tests were repeated and confirmed in less than a week. Not knowing what this all meant at the time, my estimated glomerular filtration rate (EGFR) was only 13–15, my creatinine was 4.7, and my blood urea nitrogen (BUN) was 6. In addition, just about all of my red blood cell indicators were below the normal threshold: all indicators of how poorly my kidneys were functioning. What is happening to me? In the words of the singer/songwriter Marvin Gaye, "What's Going On?" I mean what's *really, really* going on?

CHAPTER 2

Diagnosis
Who Me?

Let me start by saying I am a patient; I am not a doctor. Like most things in life, experiences vary from person to person; this is *my* experience.

It has been said that an accurate diagnosis is half the cure. As a child, my "feelings" were hurt so often that over time, I became slow to even recognize physical discomfort or pain—save that drama for your mama, grin and bear it. The 80/20 rule: 80% of people don't care, and the other 20% are glad it's *not* happening to them, including some who delight in your demise.

During my school days, I took a health science course, and I recall the professor cautioning us during one of his lectures about maintaining our health by forming good habits in our youth. I remember him saying something to the effect of, "Maintenance is cheaper than repair." No truer words were ever spoken. Hundred-dollar bill, Benjamin Franklin, said it this way, "An ounce of prevention is worth a pound of cure."

Actually, my declining health story began much sooner than January 2022. I recall being very sick (like never before sick) in the last week of 2019, spilling over into the first week of the new year. I remember taking over-the-counter medicines and even trying to sweat out the virus at my local gym—remember, I didn't have health insurance at that time, so I was reluctant to go to the emergency room. My sister finally convinced me to seek professional medical help, so I visited the Patient First clinic near my home.

Barely being able to sit up straight and cough without having a stinging pain in my lower back, the clinicians did the usual and asked me for my insurance card—first things first. I informed them that I did not have insurance and that I would self-pay. After collecting my payment information and a copy of my driver's license, they then sent me back for medical observation. They took my weight, my temperature, and my blood pressure (I took them all back before I left) and asked me about my symptoms and how long I had been feeling bad. They then proceeded to take a chest X-ray and a urine sample.

Ultimately, the physician assistant prescribed antibiotics but was concerned with my blood pressure, and urine test, and recommended I schedule an appointment with an endocrinologist and nephrologist as soon as possible. I didn't know exactly what each specialized in, so I said to myself, "I'm not going to see two doctors for one body." I decided to make an appointment with the nephrologist—primarily because the earliest I could schedule an appointment with the endocrinologist was six months out, and since I knew nothing about nephrology, I thought maybe I might learn something new. I was able to get in rather quickly to see the nephrologist.

My appointment was on January 20, 2020. It was the same routine as my Patient First visit; they wanted my insurance information, and I informed them that I did not have insurance and that I would self-pay. After collecting my payment information and a copy of my driver's license, you know the rest.

When I got back to see the doctor, he was a nice fella around my age. He interviewed me and asked what landed me here in his office, and I explained. It was a pleasant casual conversation. We both talked about where we were originally from, and I asked him why he chose this particular specialty—to be honest, I don't remember what he said, but I feigned interest because in my mind I thought I'd never be back in this place again. He asked about my line of work, and I told him I used to be in insurance but was now retired, and he replied, "I'm jealous." We both laughed, and he left the room for a bit, ostensibly to review my test results.

When he returned, we discussed the results of my blood and urine test. My HbA1c was 9.3 (normal range is 4.8–5.6). Uh oh, somebody's diabetic! My creatinine was 1.9 (normal range is .76–1.27). Oh no, somebody's kidneys aren't up to par. My BUN was 23 (normal range is 8–27), and my blood protein number was 7.8 (normal range is 6–8.5). He didn't give me a specific EGFR number at the time but told me I was in stage 3 out of 5 CKD (chronic kidney disease). When the doctor stepped out of the office a second time, I peeked at my medical record on the computer screen.

The electronic records showed that in July of 2014 (the last time I had a PCP), my EGFR was 95 if of African descent but 82 if otherwise—I'll explain this farcical discrepancy a little later down the line. I asked the nephrologist if there was any way I could improve from stage 3 and get back to stage 1. He stated that was not possible but what I could do is try to maintain my current functionality and do some things to slow down the progression of the disease. He advised me to be cognizant of my sodium consumption, stop taking anti-inflammatory meds apart from aspirin, increase my water intake, and follow up in two months. He also prescribed blood pressure medicine—which was already prescribed by the physician assistant at Patient First. I didn't notice any major changes in how I felt, so I said, "Thanks for the advice," and went on my merry way.

But even as far back as 2011, I had a pre-diabetes diagnosis in which my HbA1c (a blood test that indicates how much glucose/sugar on average is in your blood over a ninety-day timeframe) was around 6.4%. Because the normal HbA1c range is 4.8% to 5.6%, one is considered to have pre-diabetes if their number is between 5.7–6.4%, and if the number is greater than 6.4%, the person is a diabetic.

I became vegan and more consistent with my exercise routine and lost about thirty pounds. I was retested about six months later, and my number had fallen to 5.5%. *Who needs medicine?* I began to believe—*big* mistake.

When I think back on it, my blood pressure had been high since my early thirties. I would often be asked by medical professionals, including dentists, if my blood pressure was normally elevated. I would respond by saying, "I don't know. I don't think so."

And the doctors would blow it off with a joke-like comment. "Well, it must be white coat syndrome."

Anyway, back to 2020: roughly a month after my Patient First visit, I started hearing about this strange respiratory virus that originated in China, and cases had started to appear on the West Coast of the United States. Aha! That must be why I was so sick at the end of the year! Denial is not just a river in Egypt; it's long and deep too.

An old buddy of mine from Los Angeles was in town for a congressional Black Caucus meeting in Washington, DC. It was the first week of February, and he stayed at my home for a couple of days. He was hoarding toilet paper and talked about shortages and buying restrictions on certain items in California that were not in place on the East Coast yet.

About a month later, on a Wednesday night, March 11, 2020, to be exact, I was watching a professional basketball game on television. The game stopped midway through, and the stadium was evacuated. I remember jumping up immediately and going to the grocery store to stock up—this had to be serious if a major sporting event was canceled! I called my children, who lived out of town, and recommended that they do the same. COVID-19 was in full effect! Many lives would be lost worldwide, and life as we knew it was about to change dramatically.

The pandemic caused such widespread panic that practically every corner of society was majorly affected. Businesses were either forced to close or offered restricted services, including doctor's offices. In the early stages of the pandemic, individuals (including myself) were reluctant to congregate in public places or interact with strangers—with a special aversion to sick people. In my mind, I wasn't sick, so I couldn't take the chance of being around those who were.

Although the isolation and panic caused by the pandemic took their toll on society, I enjoyed the solitude and overall deceleration of the fast-spinning world. I had lots of travel plans post my July 2019 retirement, but all those plans had to be readjusted. The spring and summer of that year allowed me to slow down and appreciate the simple things in life. I started taking nature walks and just walking in my neighborhood for hours. I had lived here for years but knew very few street names because I was usually zooming by in my car on my way to someplace else.

I had health insurance now, so I returned to Patient First as a follow-up to my January appointment earlier that year. I had been walking, hiking, and riding my bike for about three months at this juncture, so my glucose level and blood pressure had slightly improved, and I don't recall the same alarmist reaction shown in January from the physician assistant at this visit.

In the past, I rarely read fiction books, electing instead to spend my *casual* reading time on business-related subjects or nonfiction—just the facts, ma'am, just the facts. But my appetite changed, and I read maybe ten to twelve fiction books as well as the usual six to eight nonfiction offerings over the next year to year and a half.

On October 3, I felt really bad after returning from a two-and-a-half-hour walk through the neighborhood and a wooded park that I had grown fond of approximately three miles from my home. I don't remember drinking any water while out that day, and it was a relatively warm day for that time of year. Once I made it home, I drank some water, took a hot shower, and lay down for what I thought would be a quick nap—it was early, maybe seven or seven thirty that evening.

When I woke up the next morning, my right wrist and elbow were both swollen, and I had a sharp pain in the center left of my upper back. I had difficulty leveraging myself to get out of bed or lift myself off the couch. I thought this would pass, but the swelling didn't subside, and I progressively felt worse. Again, my sister strongly suggested that I seek medical help; after all, it had been a week, and things weren't getting better.

It took me about two hours to sit up and get dressed before I was able to drive myself to my go-to medical facility, Patient First. This time, they advised me to go to the emergency room immediately. My daughter, who was in residency at Georgetown Hospital in Washington, DC, drove up to take me to the emergency room and insisted I go to Johns Hopkins Hospital located about twenty miles from my neighborhood as opposed to the local hospital because she wanted me to get the best possible care.

I was admitted and went through a battery of tests for four days. I felt better upon discharge, but I did not get a clear understanding of what was wrong with me. A side note: I had to have a COVID test before being admitted or assigned to a room and no visitors—this was protocol back then.

My discharge papers showed that I may have had pseudo-gout—another sign that there's a problem with filtering toxins from my body. They suggested I start seeing a PCP regularly and went so far as to put me in touch with one near my home. This was top-shelf treatment, and I was so moved that I wrote the hospital a letter expressing my gratitude for getting me back on my feet. In addition, I was officially diagnosed as a diabetic and encouraged to work with my PCP to manage my blood glucose and blood pressure. What they did not tell me was my EGFR was only around 30 even back then.

I began seeing the PCP on October 28 and saw her again in November and December of 2020. My final visit with her was in May of 2021. There was a concerted effort to lower my blood pressure, blood glucose, and cholesterol, which had skyrocketed to 346 (it's recommended that this number be kept under 200). I was prescribed three blood pressure medicines, a statin for my cholesterol, as well as a daily dose of baby aspirin—81 milligrams.

I was finally able to see an endocrinologist in May or June of 2021. He was my age and shared that he too was diabetic. He commented that I had pretty good control of my glucose (which I was controlling via diet and exercise) and recommended that I continue to limit my carbohydrate intake, meaning no more than 60 grams per meal. That seemed generous based on my eating habits at that time. I mentioned that I never had problems with my cholesterol level in the past and wondered why it was out of whack. I remember him saying, "Once one organ starts to go bad, it's like a chain reaction."

He also recommended that the common drug used by doctors to manage diabetes in most patients (metformin) should be avoided at all costs because it is metabolized by the kidneys and would lead to kidney failure in six months or less. That seemed melodramatic or hyperbolic to me, so I said, "Okay, I'm managing my diabetes with diet and exercise. I'm not big on medicine anyway."

I also stopped taking the cholesterol medicine that spring because it caused cramping in my hands, legs, and feet, at least that's what I thought and maybe it did, but kidneys also balance the body's fluid (water) and electrolytes (sodium, calcium, potassium, and phosphate to name a few), so this could have been yet another indicator of my declining kidney function. Again, denial is not just a river in Egypt.

I want to give you this background information because I am often asked by people if there were any early warning signs that my kidneys were failing or that I had chronic kidney disease. Because I appeared healthy, was fairly active, and didn't live recklessly, I am asked if there was anything I could have done to stave off what ultimately led to my kidney failure? I know what they're really asking is if there is anything *they* can do to avoid this horrific fate.

In retrospect, I would encourage individuals to get annual physical exams beginning around the age of twenty-five; this will establish a baseline of health. Diseases like type 2 diabetes and hypertension tend to rear their ugly heads later in life—like love, youth has a way of covering a multitude of faults. Number two: know your family's health history; you not only inherited Grandpa's good looks and Grandma's ways; you also may have inherited their propensity for certain chronic diseases. From there, monitor and manage changes with a health professional. If your twenty-fifth birthday is a distant memory, start now!

I did not return to see the nephrologist until September 29, 2021. I was feeling more comfortable congregating in public at this time as my second COVID-19 vaccine dose was completed on May 1, 2021. Although I did not feel bad, things had gotten much worse by the time I returned for my nephrology follow-up visit. A nurse once told me, "You get used to feeling a certain way, but that doesn't mean you're okay."

In actuality, I had started to notice some changes. I would joke with my friends that I would wake up today and go to bed tomorrow—that no matter what time I went to bed, I would sleep no more than five hours. For example, if I went to bed at 10:00 p.m., I'd wake up at 2:00 or 3:00 a.m., so I started to go to bed "tomorrow," around 1:30 or 2:00 a.m. so that I'd wake up around 6:00 or 7:00 a.m. I did not know it at the time, but this too is another symptom of kidney problems.

I was napping during the day, nodding out like a heroin junkie if I sat still too long, and by December, I was urinating every two hours at night—I would later learn the term for this is nocturia, which in my case was yet another sign of my declining kidney function. I could hear my pulse rapidly pounding in my temples when I lay down to go to sleep at night—blood pressure issues—and my urine was so foamy, it looked like the suds you see when pouring out warm beer or bubbles like that bubble-blowing game played by children (maybe not that sudsy or bubbly but close). I was leaking protein in my urine, which is medically known as proteinuria.

In a little over a year and a half, my blood test indicators were below the normal thresholds. My BUN was way above normal, my creatinine had gone from 1.9 (not good) to 2.73, and my EGFR had fallen to 25. With each new blood test, my results just kept getting worse. My potassium, weight, cholesterol, blood pressure, and blood glucose were all on the rise, while my kidney function indicators were all on the decline.

Damn!

To boot, I spent the spring, summer, and fall of 2021 going back and forth with my health insurance company because they refused to pay the medical bills accumulated over the 2020 and 2021 time periods.

The reason: they stated that I did not disclose on my March 2020 application that a medical professional (Patient First) had diagnosed me with high blood pressure, leaving me stuck with over $20,000 in out-of-pocket medical expenses.

Damn! Damn!

CHAPTER 3

Reality Check/Nephro Please!

Let me start by saying I am a patient; I am not a doctor. Like most things in life, experiences vary from person to person; this is *my* experience.

So after paying health insurance premiums for eighteen months, here I was again with no health insurance because my policy had been rescinded (meaning canceled as if it were never in effect) and my premiums were returned—six months later I might add. After all these years, I was finally starting to need and use health insurance in a meaningful way for myself, and I was without it for 2020 and 2021. What to do?

At the time, I was under the age of fifty-nine and unable to access my 401K without penalty, and when you couple that with the fact that I had no income, I decided to apply for Medicaid in my state as my frequent visits to the doctor were eating away at my savings. I qualified and was granted coverage beginning in January of 2022. This was a big help as I had no idea about the medical costs I would experience in the coming year.

On February 9, 2022, I was told to report to the emergency room. I was called by the nephrology nurse—let's call her Natasha. She had a noticeable Russian accent and seemed to sing in a soprano-like voice when she spoke.

I remember being at the gas station when I received that call, and I asked, "Who me? What's the problem? I've got things to do!" She was very coy in her response but encouraged me to go to the emergency room as soon as possible—but no later than today. I agreed and went on to finish what I was doing and checked in at the hospital later that afternoon; they ended up keeping me there for two days. The results from my January 22nd and 27th blood test showed that my EGFR was less than 15 even with the added points for those of African descent.

As mentioned in the previous chapter, EGFR if African American is the farcical calculation used to estimate kidney function differences between African Americans and everybody else. This difference was based on small sample–size studies that began in the 1970s.

Here's the background: actual GFR (glomerular filtration rate) tests are expensive and lengthy, so creatinine filtration is used to estimate how well the kidneys are doing their job in catching the bad stuff and returning the good stuff to your bloodstream. Creatinine is a by-product of muscle metabolism (breakdown) and is easily measured because it is excreted unchanged by the kidneys. If not enough is reabsorbed by the muscles and too much is left in the blood or urine, this is a good-proxy indicator that something isn't quite right with the kidneys. The normal range for creatinine is .76–1.27, and the normal range for BUN (which only measures the nitrogen part of urea in the blood) is between 8 and 27.

It's a relatively complicated calculation with coefficients or adjustments for age (makes sense), gender (makes sense), and race (nonsense). The CKD-EPI equation, expressed as a single equation, is: GFR = 141 * min(Scr/$\varkappa$,1)$^{\alpha}$ * max(Scr/$\varkappa$, 1)$^{-1.209}$ * 0.993^{Age} * 1.018 [if female] * 1.159 [if black].

Based on this small sample size back in the day, researchers concluded that Black men and women excreted higher rates of creatinine than Whites. Researchers pontificated that Blacks have more muscle mass than Whites and therefore would have more muscle breakdown, leading to more excretion of creatinine by-product, resulting in an exaggerated reading, and because of this, sixteen to twenty-one percentage points needed to be added back to the EGFR. No consideration was given for body type, genetic history, diet, lifestyle, or existing diseases—ridiculous!

The inflated EGFR has led to incorrect or late chronic disease diagnoses for millions of people over the past half century. Think about it, this could mean a misdiagnosis of a person's CKD stage, which dictates treatment, medication, referrals, and even transplantation listing. For example, in my 2014 chart, my EGFR was 82, but because I identify as a Black American, the 1.16 coefficient was applied, and my filtration rate appeared to be 95. I left the doctor's office feeling confident about my kidney function when in fact the decline had already begun.

Imagine someone who has an EGFR of 28, which is stage 4 (right at the doorstep of kidney failure) and was told that the number would be multiplied by 1.16 or 1.21 because they are of African descent. One would be led to believe their kidney function was four to six points higher respectively or stage 3b of the disease—crazy!

In fact, muscle mass can't even be measured by simply eyeballing someone; an X-ray, CT scan, or the like is needed for a truly accurate measurement—shameful!

According to the US Census Bureau website, the 1997 Office of Management and Budget (OMB) set the standard for race and ethnicity in the United States and its territories. There are five categories to choose from—White, Black or African American, American Indian or Alaska Native, Asian, and Native Hawaiian or Other Pacific. An individual's response to a race question is based upon self-identification and beginning in the year 2000 individuals were allowed to report more than one race on the US Census form. Race is a social construct used primarily for government policymaking decisions but has absolutely nothing to do with anatomy or biology at its core. While there may be certain social or cultural norms and traditions practiced by a particular population subgroup there is no fundamental difference in the human race. In fact, a so-called White person could be more genealogically aligned with a so-called Black person than they are with another White and vice versa, but I digress.

Thankfully, the medical profession is slowly moving away from this false distinction.

The two equations for EGFR predominate in North American health-care systems are the 1999 Modification of Diet in Renal Disease (MDRD) equation and the 2009 Chronic Kidney Disease Epidemiology Collaboration (CKD-EPI). EGFR measures the level of creatinine in your blood—the higher the creatinine level in the blood, the more likely a person has CKD. What's also being measured is how quickly your blood is filtered per minute and if the creatinine is being reabsorbed into your bloodstream. EGFR is often spoken about in percentages because it's easier to comprehend when thought of as a percentage of function.

Chronic kidney disease is measured in five stages, which are calculated using EGFR. The stages are as follows: stage 1 indicates that a person's kidneys are properly filtering greater than or equal to 90% of waste products found in the blood; stage 2 indicates 60–89% filtration rate; stage 3 is divided into two sections—3a indicating 45–59% and 3b 30–44% filtration rate; stage 4 indicates 15–29%; and stage 5, which is kidney failure, means your kidneys are functioning at less than 15% of capacity, excreting proteins and leaving an excessive amount of the waste/toxins circulating throughout your body.

Chronic Kidney Disease Stages	
Classification	EGFR
Stage 1	≥90
Stage 2	60–89
Stage 3a	45–59
Stage 3b	30–44
Stage 4	15–29
Stage 5	<15

According to the Centers for Disease Control and Prevention (the CDC), non-Hispanic Black adults represent 20% of chronic kidney disease patients. That's disproportionate considering "Blacks" make up approximately 12–13% of the US population, and when you take into account that nine out of ten people are unaware that they even have kidney disease, the 20% number is more than likely underestimated.

The nephrologist wasn't quite sure why my kidney function was declining so rapidly and wanted to do a renal and bladder ultrasound to determine if I had suffered an acute injury to either organ. The results showed that there was no acute injury from a car accident, a boxing match, or any rough-and- tumble contact sport, just plain, old-fashioned chronic abuse.

On March 16, 2022, Natasha called a second time, this time informing me that it was official; I had end-stage renal disease (ESRD), meaning my kidney function was below fifteen percent, and to schedule a follow-up visit in six weeks to discuss my options.

Options? What? Have both of my kidneys failed? You mean to tell me that I don't have at least one good kidney left? Can't you just remove the bad one? Are you sure? What the!

Please say it ain't so! They explained that kidneys are interdependent or interconnected and one cannot exist without the other—when one goes bad, they both go bad—they are not mutually exclusive. Although a person can live with only one kidney, such as the case with a healthy living donor, kidneys fail simultaneously. There is no good kidney or bad kidney in chronic kidney disease.

Okay, this is serious—duh? My new nephrologist and Natasha had my full attention. I wanted to know everything they knew about kidneys and, more specifically, what my options were.

Full transparency—I didn't know much about kidneys. Sure, I had heard of this organ and knew there was a bean named after it, and when I watched boxing matches, I would hear the announcer talk about kidney punches, but I had no idea how important this organ was to one's overall good health. I guess nothing *really* matters until it matters to you.

Some of my initial findings were that the kidneys are a pair of bean-shaped organs located on either side of the spine—one on the right and the other on the left side. The kidneys are protected by back muscle and fat—the upper two-thirds also are protected by the lower rib cage.

Each kidney weighs about five ounces, about the same as a baseball, an apple, or a cell phone, and contains approximately one million filtering units called nephrons. Thus, a kidney doctor is called a nephrologist.

Each nephron is made of a glomerulus (pronounced *glo-meer-you-lus*) and a tubule (pronounced *too-byool*). The glomerulus is likened to a sieve or sifter, and the tubule is like a tube connected to the glomerulus. The kidneys are connected to the urinary bladder by tubes called ureters. Urine is stored in the urinary bladder until the bladder is emptied by urinating. The bladder is connected to the outside of the body by another tube-like structure called the urethra, located in the male or female organ.

I asked the nephrologist what other resources or reading materials were available for me to learn more about kidneys and their function. I was referred to the National Kidney Foundation, the American Kidney Fund, the National Institute of Health, and the DaVita websites. I also referenced my home edition of *Anatomica* and scoured the Internet for videos and any additional information I could find regarding kidney function, dysfunction, and treatments—here's an amalgamation of what I learned.

What are kidneys, and what exactly do they do?

The human body has about six quarts of blood that is constantly being circulated all day every day throughout your body for as long as you live. Okay, but tell me about the kidneys. Kidneys are regulators and filters. On average, a person circulates about fifty gallons of blood (a fluid made of red and white blood cells, platelets, and plasma) a day. Your kidneys filter all of that, ridding your blood of salt, excess water, and toxic waste, which is then passed on to your bladder as urine. Of the fifty gallons filtered per day, about one-half gallon or two quarts are peed out during the day. Meanwhile, the clean blood is returned to the heart, and the entire process starts all over again. It's starting to make sense why I've heard since I was a child to drink eight cups of water a day—eight cups equal a half gallon, and this amount helps in flushing your kidneys.

The kidneys also release hormones that regulate blood pressure, manage the body's overall fluid balance, and help in managing vitamin D absorption, which aids in balancing the calcium and phosphorous in your body. This is crucial for bone health by regulating the parathyroid hormone (PTH) so that it does not send the wrong signal to the glands that the body needs additional calcium. If this happens, the body starts looking for calcium anywhere it can find it and starts to pull calcium from the bones (including teeth), making them weak. So it's not milk that gives you strong bones? Hmmm.

Normal kidneys and kidney function

Chronic kidney disease means your kidneys are damaged and have lost their ability to keep you healthy by filtering your blood. In the early stages of the disease, most people do not have symptoms. But as kidney disease gets worse, waste can build up in your blood and make you feel sick. This is what happened to me. I had no idea my kidney function had been on the decline over the past ten years because I was active; believed I had decent, if not good, dietary habits; and didn't recognize the symptoms early in the disease.

You may also develop other kidney problems, like high blood pressure (check), anemia (check), weak bones, poor nutritional health, and nerve damage—I would say a stroke, mini or not, qualifies as nerve damage (check).

Because kidneys are vital to so many of the body's functions, kidney disease also increases your risk of having heart and blood vessel disease, aka a stroke or heart attack.

While these problems may happen slowly and without symptoms, they can lead to kidney failure, which can appear without warning. This was my experience and the experience of millions of others and, unfortunately, will be the experience for millions more. Per the National Kidney Foundation, kidney disease affects an estimated thirty-seven million people in the United States (15% of the adult population; more than one in seven adults). And as mentioned earlier, nine in ten American adults who have kidney disease don't know it, not to mention the one in three who are unaware that they have serious chronic kidney disease.

Once kidneys fail, dialysis or a kidney transplant is needed to stay alive.

In terms of who or what ethnic group is more prone (not exclusively) to this disease, American Blacks suffer kidney failure at a higher rate than any other racially identified group. According to the American Kidney Fund, more than one in three kidney failure patients in the United States are Black. This is primarily due to the increased rates of diabetes and high blood pressure—the leading causes of kidney disease and failure.

According to the American Kidney Fund, diabetes and high blood pressure affect Blacks differently than other races. Around 12% of Blacks have diabetes, and a whopping 55% of Black adults have high blood pressure according to the American Heart Association. Please don't misunderstand. These two ailments are not exclusive to any one racial group, but American Blacks are more likely to experience kidney failure due to these ailments than other racially identified groups.

Uncontrolled diabetes (high glucose levels in the blood) is the number one cause of kidney failure, and hypertension/high blood pressure is the second highest cause. There are other less common reasons for kidney failure, but those are not my experience, so I won't discuss them here.

The American Kidney Fund has reported that in the last thirty-five years, the number of people with diabetes has doubled. It's been said repeatedly that Americans have poor eating habits. That's a bit dismissive in my opinion for a country with such abundance. I would characterize it this way: most Americans have unconscious eating habits.

What is diabetes? People often use euphemisms to describe this deadly disease by using terms like "My sugar is running high today," "I got the sugar," "she's just a little sweet," or "he's acting strange today, his sugar must be high." High blood sugar is not a treat; it's a *major health concern*!

The best explanation I've heard about what diabetes is came from a nurse years ago. We eat and drink calories to provide energy and nutrition to our bodies. Despite what the menu or advertisers say, there are only three types of food: proteins, fats, and carbohydrates. Carbohydrates supply the quickest form of energy, followed by proteins and then fat—meaning, they are released slower into your bloodstream.

The pancreas naturally produces the hormone insulin and releases it when you consume carbohydrates. Insulin acts as a key that unlocks your cells so that the carbs/glucose can be absorbed into the cells for quick energy. When your cells become resistant to insulin or insulin resistant, your pancreas keeps producing insulin, eventually overloading your system with too much insulin until it no longer produces enough. When this happens, the glucose floats in your bloodstream and turns into fat—usually stored in your body in all the wrong places. But beyond cosmetics, this sugary concoction circulates through your body, wreaking havoc on your organs—especially the kidneys, whose job is to filter all that filthy blood.

Hypertension or high blood pressure is also underestimated in similar ways as high blood sugar. The medical profession uses enigmatic terms like *silent killer* all while telling you this with a facial expression incongruent with what you were just told about your impending *death*. And individuals talk about their blood pressure as something akin to someone or something irritating them: "Ooh wee you gettin' on my nerves, you makin' my pressure rise." Imagine sucking and blowing liquid through a straw with no obstruction, and then try the same suction and blowing motion while pinching the straw—your jaws feel the difference. Multiply this by the millions of vessels in your body.

As the saying goes, "Pressure busts pipes," and blood vessels too.

CHAPTER 4

Information Overload

Let me start by saying I am a patient; I am not a doctor. Like most things in life, experiences vary from person to person; this is *my* experience.

I must admit I was overwhelmed when I received the news that my kidneys were well on their way to shutting down completely—more than tongue can tell. I've shared those deep feelings with my pillow, and it has absorbed all the stories I could never tell another. Eventually, I shared my diagnosis with five other people: my two children, my two bookend siblings (older brother and younger sister), and a relatively new friend that I had grown close to. Truth be told, I was embarrassed, ashamed, disappointed in myself, and stymied by the fear of the unknown.

Even in revealing my diagnosis to those individuals, I downplayed my concerns—but my daughter and sister (who is a hospital pharmacist) had a better understanding of what lay ahead for me. You know, embarrassment tends to harbor a tinge of resentment or anger, and disappointment harbors sorrow and sadness, but shame begets repentance. I decided to lean into the shame and commit to changing for the better and maybe, just maybe, become a shining example of how to deal with tough times for others who receive devastating health news.

Behind the scenes, the nephrologist had forwarded my information to DaVita, Inc., a company headquartered in Denver, Colorado, and one of the leaders in kidney dialysis services. I had seen DaVita signs in cities I lived in over the years but never knew exactly what service or product the company provided. The name DaVita is actually derived from the Italian phrase *Dare Vita*, which means "giving life." I later learned that one of their competitors is a company by the name of Fresenius. I had never heard of them prior to being on dialysis and only found out about them from one of the DaVita technicians while discussing her job options.

DaVita and Fresenius dominate the dialysis market accounting for more than 80% of centers nationwide and have a pipeline into most nephrology practices across the country. By late March, at the request of the nephrologist, I scheduled an in-person class with Kidney Smart—a DaVita-affiliated organization designed to educate patients and their caregivers about treatment options, diet, insurance coverage, and the transplant process.

There are two main types of dialysis. Both types filter your blood to rid your body of harmful wastes, extra salt, and water: hemodialysis or peritoneal dialysis. The other non-dialysis option was conservative care, which I had no interest in pursuing. Conservative care is hospice, pain management, and fading to black. I wasn't willing to give up just yet without a fight.

The educators were well versed in the subject matter, but it was way too much information, maybe not for the *well me* but too much for the *sick me*. They asked me if I lived alone or with someone. I answered, "Alone." Then they went on to ask if I preferred hemodialysis or peritoneal dialysis, if I preferred to receive my dialysis in a dialysis facility, or if would I prefer to do it myself at home. What! Then the educator showed me the machine I would use if I chose the at-home option. They would train me for two weeks on how to use the machine if I decided to move forward with home dialysis. Huh? Two weeks!

Peritoneal required having a tube installed in my abdomen, like a three-to-five-inch pull cord (like a talking doll) protruding from my stomach that I would use to connect to the machine. The dialysis fluid (connected to the machine) would clean my blood overnight as I slept—every night. Boxes of fluid would be delivered to my home I think on a biweekly or monthly basis. It seemed their only concern was if I had enough space in my home or garage to store twenty or thirty huge boxes of fluid. *My concern was how the heck could I carry one box, let alone twenty-plus boxes in my now-weakened state. Supposedly a majority of nephrologists would choose this option—oh, really?*

The other at-home option is hemodialysis. A smaller version of the machine used in a dialysis center is given to the patient to take home. These brave souls do four to five home treatments a week for three-and-a-half to four hours—inserting the needles into their arms themselves (self-cannulation) or by a trusted family member or friend caregiver.

Peritoneal is frightening enough but is basically a fluid concoction flushing your system through osmosis. Hemodialysis involves needles and blood—knowing the difference between veins and arteries, *yikes*.

I discussed the options with my daughter, and she advised hemodialysis was the best option due to concerns about infection associated with peritoneal treatments.

Now that that was settled, I needed to decide if I wanted to do in-center day treatments three-and-a-half to four hours three times a week or nocturnal dialysis—overnight treatment's eight hours a night, three times a week. There are pros and cons to both options, but I knew I did not want to sleep in a chair at a facility three nights a week.

I thought to myself that maybe my luck had run out and my time was up—I had to remind myself of one of my lifelong mottos: "Don't cry the blues when you lose. Keep the same grin when you win."

I discussed my hesitation with my daughter and friend about moving forward with treatment. My friend put me in touch with her nephew who had been on dialysis for two years before receiving a transplant a year and a half prior to our conversation. I explained my situation and concerns to him. He could relate because he had firsthand knowledge of the journey I was contemplating. He shared his story with me and was very encouraging, which gave me some hope. He was actually in Mexico at the time enjoying himself poolside when we spoke—at that point in my sickness, I could only imagine.

It was now April, and I had been in end-stage renal failure for approximately four months—a decision needed to be made ASAP.

As mentioned before, I had scoured the Internet for videos and listened to scores of so-called gurus and their sound advice on how to heal yourself naturally and avoid dialysis. This sound advice turned out to be ninety-five percent sound and five percent advice.

The kicker for me was my brief but spectacular conversation with my daughter. She simply said, "Dad, if you want to live, you have no choice."

I decided to move forward with in-center hemodialysis treatment. From that day forward, I vowed to see this thing through, regardless of the outcome.

The ultimate goal was to receive a transplant. The waiting period in Maryland for a deceased donor was approximately two to five years. I could easily do two maybe three years on a waitlist. I've stayed committed to situations I had limited interest in much longer than that.

Dating as far back as my high school and college-basketball-playing days, if I've heard it once, I've heard it a hundred times: "Son, you see a lot, you see nothing. You see a little, you see everything. Don't worry about climbing the mountain in the distance, deal with the pebble in your shoe." Focus man, focus!

I know that commitment is a muscle and just like any other muscle, it has to be exercised. I vowed to have perfect attendance with my dialysis treatments come hell or high water!

Now I needed to have outpatient surgery to have a central venous catheter placed in my chest—this allows for dialysis to begin almost immediately and is a temporary way to administer the dialysis fluid and blood flow until a more permanent fistula or graft access can surgically be inserted in the arm and allowed to mature, usually in six to eight weeks.

In hindsight, I probably should have scheduled the fistula operation back in February or March and avoided the need for a catheter operation, but hindsight is 20/20. A fistula is a surgical procedure that connects a vein and artery to create a large thick vein under the skin to do the job the catheter was doing but more efficiently with less risk of infection.

My catheter operation was on Thursday, May 5, 2022, at Dialysis Access Specialists in Timonium, Maryland. The preferred placement of the catheter is on the right side of the chest, farthest away from one's heart just below the clavicle bone.

By this time, I was noticeably different. It's as if once I was diagnosed, my symptoms came on rapidly—a kind of Pygmalion effect. I had no appetite, and just about anything I ate left a metallic taste on my tongue; my breathing was more labored, and my energy level had dramatically declined—red blood cell production was way down. I had lost about twenty pounds since my January doctors' appointments, and my urination was less frequent—but again I wasn't consuming much liquid because of the taste, further dehydrating myself. Periodically, I would vomit a yellowish or light-green bile usually in the mornings or have excessive coughing spells, also most times in the morning.

My estimated kidney function at this point was below 10%—I was in bad shape!

My daughter took me to the early-morning outpatient surgery appointment that was scheduled to take no more than an hour. After the procedure, I passed out and was taken to the Greater Baltimore Medical Center Emergency Room, this time via an ambulance. I had never been in an ambulance before in my life. Although I regained consciousness shortly after passing out, the medical professionals insisted I go to the emergency room via emergency medical technicians (EMTs). I was anemic, and my blood pressure would drop upon standing. I was admitted to the hospital that morning but didn't get a room until around 9:00 p.m. I was administered my first dialysis treatment in the hospital on Friday, May 6, via my newly placed catheter.

The first time I fainted was in the barber's chair back in February—scared the bejesus out of my barber and the other patrons. I recovered after about ten minutes (just in time before the EMTs arrived) and assured everyone that I was okay before driving myself home. At that time, I thought it was because I hadn't eaten all day, which was becoming pretty common during this period.

I was released from the hospital on Saturday, May 7, and was driven home by an Uber driver. This was my first solo Uber ride, and it was paid for by my health insurance—lots of firsts that weekend. My daughter returned to work that Thursday afternoon as she had only expected to be away from the office for a few hours that morning for what we believed to be a simple catheter insertion procedure.

During May and again in early June, I had to have an echocardiogram and a stress test. The goal was to prove my heart was healthy enough to have the arteriovenous fistula surgery (the abnormal connection between an artery and a vein described above), which is placed in the bicep of the left arm, or if your heart is strong enough, it's inserted in the forearm. The stronger the heart, the closer to the wrist area. The surgeon must leave room to move up the arm as blood flow decreases over time—in the words of the cartoon character Charlie Brown, "Good Grief!" Also, the vein expands due to the increased blood flow, and you can actually feel the throbbing pulsation of blood flow in your arm.

I had a pre-surgery appointment with the surgeon's office about a week before my surgery. The purpose of this visit was to map the artery and vein location in my left arm to calculate the best placement of the fistula—the arm closest to my heart. At this point, I felt like I was either going to dialysis or going to doctors' appointments.

My surgeon only performed fistula operations on Tuesdays. I had the option of having mine done on June 21 or July 5. My daughter was advocating for me to have the operation done sooner rather than later as catheters are prone to infection, so I was instructed to not get mine wet—in other words, no sweating and, yes, no showers.

Allow me to tell you a little bit about my daughter. My daughter was born the day before my birthday. What a wonderful birthday gift! She was supposed to come before me! Now here she was, looking after me, taking me to my appointments, and advising me on my health care.

When she was a baby, I remember thinking I would do all I could to see that she would grow up to be the type of woman I'd be proud of one day. I was so nervous but serious about that thought. I can hardly keep the buttons on my shirt nowadays—Dr. J, my Miss Jorie (who came into the world and changed my life).

My siblings had been planning a family reunion a year earlier and agreed to have it on the weekend of June 18–21. The last family reunion I took part in was nine years earlier, and there seemed to be a necessity as our family members were getting older and COVID restrictions had limited travel and interaction with one another for the past two years. So I agreed to be involved nine months before I knew about my health problems.

I remember having a conversation with my son about the upcoming surgery and not attending the family reunion, and his advice was as follows: "The whole point in getting treatment is so you can feel better so you can do the things you love. Pops, you decide, but if I were you, I would go."

I scheduled my surgery for the latter of the two dates and attended the family reunion.

I had a dream around this time in which my deceased mother appeared. She looked a lot younger than I remember; actually, she looked younger than me. She walked through the empty school cafeteria and passed by the table where my sister and I sat. She confidently said to me, "Everything will be all right," and kept on walking. From that day on, I knew no matter the outcome, I would indeed be all right.

My operation took place early Tuesday morning on July 5, 2022. Again, my daughter was there for me.

I had been on dialysis for only about six weeks at that time and wondered how I could travel out of town and not jeopardize my health. I discussed this with the powers that be at my DaVita Dialysis Center and was informed that it was indeed possible to travel while on dialysis. I was put in touch with DaVita Guest Services. In general, it is recommended that you plan your trip at least two weeks in advance. Once I knew when and where I was going, I contacted guest services to inform them of my destination and my desired length of stay, and they handled the rest by securing a chair at the nearest available center—not necessarily the closest because there may not be availability at the nearest location. After the location was secured, my home center forwarded my treatment plan to the destination facility along with my insurance information of course; a time was scheduled, and that was it. I was all set to spend three days in the mountains near Gatlinburg, Tennessee.

I planned to have my regular dialysis treatment on Friday, drive to Tennessee on Saturday, and have my treatment at the visiting facility on Monday before returning home on Tuesday to resume my treatment at my home facility on Wednesday. Great plan, right? Well, you know what they say about the best-made plans.

All was going as planned until the third day. My treatment was reserved at the DaVita Center in Maryville, Tennessee, about forty miles from our vacation cabin. My scheduled time was 11:00 a.m., so I expected my treatment to end around 2:30 p.m., giving me plenty of time to return to the cabin before leaving for our banquet, which was scheduled to begin around 6:00 p.m.

I left the cabin at nine that morning, giving myself enough time to get lost and still make my reservation. I told my family members who inquired that I had to take care of some business in Knoxville but would be back in plenty of time. Only two of my siblings knew the real deal, and they were sworn to secrecy.

Although it was only forty miles away from the cabin, it took about an hour and a half to arrive because the route was through the hilly backroads of the good ol' volunteer state—but I was still on schedule. There was some confusion with the paperwork, so I wasn't seated until noon. Again, I had only been on dialysis for five or six weeks at this time, so whatever. Whoo-sah!

The treatment didn't end until 3:30 p.m., and I had not eaten the entire day. I was feeling very weak and a bit disoriented, but I needed to get back to the cabin, and I had at least an-hour-and-a-half drive ahead of me. I arrived back at the cabin a little after 5:00 p.m., had a little snack, and quickly changed clothes to arrive at the banquet hall on time. The drive to the hall was about thirty minutes away from our location, but all was well—my secret was still safe.

We had a great time at the banquet, which lasted about two-and-a-half hours, and returned to the cabin to recap the night, snack, and prepare to play parlor games. I remember feeling a bit weak as I sat on a stool catching up with my sister-in-law before I felt this wave of heat and perspiration on my forehead (reminiscent of my previous fainting spells), and before I knew it, boom! The next thing I knew I was on the floor with the majority of my family hovering over me wondering what happened. It was just like my barbershop and post-catheter operation incidents.

Again, only three of my siblings knew that I was on dialysis at the time and were sworn to secrecy. My youngest sister was made privy to my condition about a week earlier as I thought it only right to inform her since we were making the eight-hour drive together from Maryland to Tennessee.

There was lots of speculation and concern regarding my fainting and sudden illness. I still did not want anyone to know, but my anemia was in full effect, so I had to delay my return plans another day. With the help of my sister who knew and understood my condition from the start, we drove back to Maryland on Wednesday, and I resumed my dialysis on both Thursday and my regularly scheduled Friday date at my home dialysis center.

Over the next week or two, I finally spilled the beans to my concerned family members and implored them in the words of Evita, "Don't Cry for Me Argentina." To my knowledge, they complied with my request and went back to their daily lives, challenges, trials, and tribulations.

I can't pinpoint when the effects of my January 2022 ministroke resurfaced, but around late May or sometime in June of that year, I noticed my gait had changed. When I stepped, my left foot would make a delayed slapping sound. I would later find out that this is known as common peroneal nerve compression aka foot drop. Oh boy, I'm falling apart piece by piece! My sister noticed the hitch in my step while we were on a short walk when she traveled back to Maryland with me after our family reunion. Again, she encouraged me to seek professional medical help, so I started physical therapy with ATI PT in the second half of July (after my fistula surgery on July 5; I believe around July 18 or 19).

I attended physical therapy twice a week until my insurance coverage ended for that service on September 1. I did exercises to strengthen my leg and ankle muscles, received electrode stimulation to reactivate the nerves, and was prescribed a medical AFO—an ankle/foot brace worn to help support the foot from flopping. Upon completion of my monitored physical therapy, my condition had not improved, so I thought to myself, *I guess this will be my new walk, and I'll just have to figure out ways to disguise my latest ailment.*

It was too exhausting to take the walks I had grown to love, so I wasn't getting much outside activity that summer—even on my so-called non-dialysis good days. But I did continue to do the home exercises I learned in physical therapy. I was reminded of what the apostle Paul said in 2 Corinthians 12: 8–9:

> Three times I pleaded with the Lord about this, that it should leave me. But He said to me, "My grace is sufficient for you, for My power is made perfect in weakness." Therefore, I will boast all the more gladly of my weaknesses, so that the power of Christ may rest upon me.

No more suffering in silence. The cat's out of the bag; let me embrace this thing and gird up for this journey no matter how long—no matter who's with or without me.

CHAPTER 5

Treatment
Win the Morning, Win the Day

Let me start by saying I am a patient; I am not a doctor. Like most things in life, experiences vary from person to person; this is *my* experience.

I was assigned to the DaVita Dialysis Center closest to my home, which was 2.6 miles away, but there was no *chair* immediately available, so I was placed at the second option 3.2 miles away and began my first in-center dialysis treatment on Monday, May 9, 2022. My scheduled duration time in the *chair* was three and a half hours and was to begin at 6:45 a.m. Monday, Wednesday, and Friday every week without exception. I would set my alarm for 5:55 a.m. on those days because the protocol was to arrive ten minutes before your scheduled time to ensure you were put on at the proper time—it didn't always happen that way, but that was the protocol.

Due to my proximity to the dialysis center, it took me approximately ten to twelve minutes to drive there, so leaving my home around 6:20 a.m. was more than ample to arrive on time—believe me, traffic is light at that hour of the morning, even the early birds are just finishing their worms. On my first day of reporting for in-center treatment, I was greeted by the office administrator, a feisty middle-aged woman with a kind heart beneath that tough exterior. I must admit that starting dialysis was a frightening experience for me, but she made the transition to dialysis a relative breeze. Her professionalism, competency, and can-do attitude gave me further confidence to move forward with my new reality.

I signed lots of papers, reminiscent of signing page after page at closing when buying a house. To be honest, I was so weak at that time that I wasn't sure what I was signing. I just knew it was required and needed to proceed with treatment. I later realized these were forms allowing my insurance to be billed as well as my consent to the treatment plan and, of course, the usual liability waivers and hold harmless agreement. I was given a small duffle bag, which included a set of headphones, a neck pillow, and a blanket. A blanket? It was the beginning of May, and the weather was warm in mid-spring. I soon learned that this was a valuable piece of equipment regardless of the time of year.

The first thing upon arriving is to enter the vestibule where you must ring the doorbell to be allowed to enter the lobby; there your forehead is used to take your temperature by an apparatus affixed to a wall. If your temperature is normal, you are then given a fresh face mask and buzzed to the back, where your dialysis chair awaits you. The area is a cafeteria-sized room with approximately twenty-five chairs spread six feet apart with a nursing station in the middle of the room. The dialysis chairs are placed along the four walls with an additional three or four directly behind the nursing station.

But before you take your chair, you must weigh yourself. This is to ensure that you are within range of your dry weight. Your dry weight is your weight when you first start dialysis adjusted periodically by the nephrologist—a person is usually a bit underweight when first starting dialysis because the toxins in your body tend to take away your appetite; at least that's how it was for me.

It is recommended that you not gain more than three kilograms between sessions, as it is risky to remove more water weight than that—risky meaning dehydration, cramping, low blood pressure, anemia, etc. You are also limited to no more than thirty-two ounces of liquid per day. That's four cups and includes all liquids and anything that would liquify at room temperature. That means ice cream, popsicles, or ice—you get the picture but not the pitcher, and hopefully you get the pun.

This is important for all dialysis patients but crucial for those who are no longer able to urinate. I was one of the lucky ones: I could still pee! It's funny what you take pride in when you're down but not out.

I grew up in the United States, and I think we are probably one of the last Western nations to not widely use the metric system. Only food companies, medical professionals, and drug dealers are proficient in this method of measurement—hmm, something to think about.

Well, dialysis has taught me that 1 kilogram multiplied by 2.2 equals your weight in pounds. For example, 80 kilograms equals 176 pounds, and 32 ounces is approximately 1 liter.

Once you have weighed yourself, you report this to the technician, and it is then recorded on the computer for tracking purposes. The technician then takes your standing blood pressure and records that as well—*now you may be seated.*

Shortly after that, the nurse comes along and asks you the same three questions every session: "Any nausea, vomiting, or diarrhea?" while checking your pulse and respiratory rate and listening for fluid buildup in your lungs by placing a stethoscope on your back and chest. After that, a small cup of water and the pills I was prescribed were taken—calcitriol (repletes calcium levels), vitamin D, an iron pill, and I can't recall what else was included. But I know there were some medicines we all received, and some are patient specific. Erythropoietin, which replenishes red blood cell production due to anemia, was given intravenously.

I wore only button-up shirts and no T-shirts to allow easy access to my catheter for the technicians. They would begin by first removing the gauze that was wrapped and taped around the two wires protruding from my chest and then clean/disinfect them with alcohol as well as clean my chest of the sticky residue left behind by the tape from the previous session. The two wires were different colors, one blue and the other red—blue for the artery and red for the vein. I asked the nurse, "How do you know which to connect to what on the machine?" She explained that *a* is for artery and arteries take the oxygenated blood *a* way and veins return the blood to the heart. So the wires/tubes are connected to the machine so that toxic blood goes into the dialyzer (a fluid concoction used to draw toxins from the blood) for cleansing and is returned via the other tube connected to my vein.

We would confirm how much fluid needed to be removed based on how much water weight was gained between sessions, and those details would be added to the digital record. Even if no water weight was gained, a minimum amount of fluid would need to be removed to flush the toxins out of your blood. Once the amount to be removed was agreed upon, the catheter would be connected to the machine, and the dialyzing process would begin.

After my fistula matured, I no longer dialyzed through my catheter and began dialyzing through my arm. Not all patients prefer hemodialysis via a graft or fistula and, despite the increased infection risk (as well as for their personal reasons), decide to continue treatment via their catheter or in some cases switch to the peritoneal option discussed earlier.

Having two needles stuck in and taken out of your arm every other day is not for the faint of heart—at least not initially.

Because when I say two needles, I'm not talking about the kind used when receiving a shot in the arm or having blood drawn for whatever reason. When I say having two needles stuck in your arm, think crochet needles or pin nails, one at a time—sheesh! I never got quite used to it, but it became a necessary evil. I was advised to apply a combination of 2.5% of lidocaine and prilocaine at least twenty minutes before being injected—it helped some I guess, or maybe I just tolerated it a little better over time. You know that sound you make when inhaling from your mouth with your teeth grit tight? That's what I did every time. The techs would say, "I know, I know. I'm so sorry. I'm so sorry. Breathe, breathe, Mr. Macoy!"

In the early days of treatment, my manly pride was hurt a bit because the woman sitting next to me never flinched when she was stuck. Then I learned she had been on dialysis for twenty-seven years, so this was old hat for her—pride restored, a tiny bit.

After a while, I came to look at my dialysis treatment as a part-time job and some of the staff and patients as friends and family. Here I was in a place I thought I'd never be, interacting triweekly with people I thought I'd never meet. I think of Booker T. Washington's most famous quote, "Cast Down Your Bucket Where You Are." This was my life, and I was intent on making the best of it.

I got used to seeing the patients on my row of five and the two additional patients in my line of sight. Unbeknownst to them, I affectionately referred to each by nicknames before I got to know them: Candyman (because he always had a Ziplock bag full of candy), Lumpy (because of the lumps on her arm, officially known as pseudoaneurysms. These occur because of repeated sticks over time—twenty-seven years qualify), Rudeboy (because he spoke to everyone but me initially), and 2Park For Sure (because his truck took up two parking spaces).

I no longer referred to my *chair* as such and now considered it to be my *seat*. I no longer looked at our row as death row and began to refer to it as the Rowboat—as in rowing gently down the stream, merrily, merrily, merrily, merrily, life is but a dream.

The two additional patients in my line of sight were nicknamed The Resident (because he was there when I arrived and there when I left) and the Comfort Zone (because she brought a winter coat and a comforter regardless of the season). Except for the Comfort Zone, the others were in their respective chairs when I arrived each morning, and all were taken off fifteen to twenty minutes before me—apart from the Comfort Zone and The Resident of course because it seemed he lived there.

Let me try to explain what it feels like physically being on dialysis—what it feels like during, immediately after, and in between treatments. I've heard through the years that dialysis makes a person tired, and this concern has made some people reluctant to start treatment. After the initial needlestick discussed above, there is no pain or realization that your blood is being pumped in and out of your body for three or four hours.

You have to be careful not to move your arm (in the case of a fistula) too abruptly for fear of dislodging the needles and spraying blood all over the place, but there is no pain. Most people occupy themselves by watching TV, sleeping (lots of sleeping), reading, listening to music, talking on the phone, or whatever is of interest to them. I would listen to an audio book or music to pass the time if I wasn't wrapped in my blanket napping away. Like clockwork, I would break my fast and my nap by eating a low-carb protein bar about an hour and fifteen minutes after I started dialyzing—8:00 a.m. to be exact.

If for whatever reason the machine is not operating properly, an alarm will sound, and the necessary adjustment is made by the technician. Sometimes, and this happened to me on a few occasions, if too much fluid is being removed too rapidly, it can cause dehydration, leading to painful leg cramps, but this is rare.

When it's time to be taken off the machine, an alarm sounds, notifying the technician that it's time to disconnect the patient. The two punctures are covered with gauze, and the patient is required to hold it in place until the bleeding stops or subsides—usually about five to ten minutes. After that, your arm/wound is wrapped, and you're asked if you feel good enough to stand. Once standing, your blood pressure is taken, and if all is within range, you return to the scale to weigh yourself, ideally returning to your original dry weight, and that number is once again recorded on the computer.

I was fortunate enough to drive myself to and from dialysis. Immediately after my treatment, I did not feel tired, but I did feel a kind of lightheadedness. Imagine working out three to four hours and losing four to six pounds of sweat and you're drained but not sleepy. This is what it's like having this much fluid removed without the benefit of exercise and sweat. But as my blood pressure slowly started to rise (in about an hour or two), I started to feel better. I would arrive home around 10:50 a.m. and prepare my breakfast, which consisted of two eggs, one slice of cheese, and a slice of low-carb bread.

From about noon to 1:45 p.m., I felt fairly good, but like a baby fighting sleep, no matter what I did, I would get drowsy by two o'clock and had to go to sleep—not a nap I'm talking about under the cover sleep until 6:00 p.m. I felt pretty good by this time and prepared my dinner, which I ate around 7:00 p.m. before calling it a night by 11:30 p.m. because there would be no early wake-up call tomorrow. Yay!

I considered my non-dialysis days my good days. I would complete my household chores, handle my bills or other business, and of course attend any doctor's visits I had scheduled. I would usually shut things down by 10:00 p.m. in preparation for my 5:55 a.m. wake-up call the next day, before starting the process all over again. Saturday and Sunday were my best days because I had a day and a half of recovery time, although things were cut short on Sundays in preparation for my Monday morning session.

I think there is a difference between tired and fatigued. Dialysis made me fatigued. It's like having a headache without the pain or a stuffy nose without having breathing problems. There's a numbness that presented itself in the roof of my mouth into my nasal passage and rested behind my eyes and in my forehead. Some have described it as brain fog—I guess it can be described that way. Because of my low red blood cell count and the excess fluid and toxins in my body, I would get fatigued after limited physical exertion—like being out of shape on the first day of practice or at the beginning of starting a workout routine. The difference is it never goes away.

As the treatments progressed, I definitely started to feel better but not because I was getting better. I think the rapid decline from stage 3 to stage 5, for example, is so dramatic that your body is shocked by the changes. What dialysis did for me, and I assume for others, is slow down the decline and held my kidney function steady, allowing my body to get used to this new limited functionality.

Dr. Willem Kolff is considered the father of dialysis. This young Dutch physician constructed the first dialyzer (artificial kidney) in 1943 (https://www.davita.com/treatment-services/dialysis/the-history-of-dialysis). He used sausage casings, a washing machine, and a water bath to create a device that could remove waste products from the blood. He tested it on fifteen patients, but only one survived.

The evolution of dialysis has come a long way from its early days. Dr. Kolff's machine was only used for acute kidney disease. It wasn't until the early 1960s that dialysis was available for long-term use, which is required for ESRD, and this wasn't widely available until Medicare benefits were expanded by law in 1972.

Dialysis machines are not perfect though. They can cause side effects like low blood pressure, infections, and fatigue. They also cannot replace all the functions of the kidneys, such as producing hormones and regulating fluids and electrolytes.

But dialysis is definitely a lifesaver or should I say a life extender for those of us with limited to no kidney function. A person with properly functioning kidneys is cleaning their blood and modulating fluid balance twenty-four hours a day seven days a week compared to dialysis for three-and-a-half hours a day three times a week.

Although dialysis is only doing roughly 10–15% of what fully functioning kidneys do, something is better than nothing, or as I like to say, it's better than a stick in the eye.

CHAPTER 6

Upside to the Downside

Let me start by saying I am a patient; I am not a doctor. Like most things in life, experiences vary from person to person; this is *my* experience.

Some people are taught to complain and unfortunately get so good at it that that's all they do. As the old Johnny Mercer lyrics explain, "You got to ac-cent-tchu-ate the positive and e-lim-inate the negative."

My life has been a barrel of blessings with a bucket of disappointments—a small bucket at that. Early in my career, I used to fly a lot, and I began to notice that no matter what the weather was on the ground, the sun was always shining above the clouds. No matter how gloomy things appeared, if I could just get above the clouds, I'm always looking to frame what happens to me in its proper light. My goal is to live in that comfortable space between elation and misery, then and next—it keeps me focused on the here and now because today is tomorrow's yesterday and yesterday's tomorrow.

As mentioned before, my dialysis days started before sunrise. Very few things rival the beauty of early morning. With its burnt-orange eastern sky loaded with layers of low puffy stratocumulus clouds in spring and summer or mystical constellations in fall and winter, it is truly a sight to behold.

The staff at my center was truly wonderful! Typically, there were two nurses, a dietician (who provided nutrition advice and biweekly reports on PTH, calcium, phosphorous, albumin, and sodium levels to name a few), and five or six technicians on duty at all times. There was a social worker who visited weekly to check on the patient's overall well-being as well as furnishing information on available social services.

My social worker was a young woman named Chekana. She was smart and knowledgeable about Social Security, Medicare, Medicaid, and other available social services. She spoke with me about these services the first week I started dialysis at the center—she got me off to a great start by supplying me with and guiding me through a myriad of forms including sending them to the proper agencies on my behalf.

Chekana is the person who explained the *Xs* and *Os* of qualifying for a deceased donor transplant and started the process of getting me listed on the waitlist at three transplant centers/hospitals. The funny thing is that I thought her name was Chakandra, and I would call her by that name in our conversations, and she never corrected me. She ended up leaving the company about seven or eight months after my meeting her, and no, it wasn't because I butchered her name but for a better employment opportunity. She was a godsend in those early days of understanding the services available to dialysis patients and navigating the multitude of paperwork associated with those services.

The nephrology nurse (Natasha) would come by once or twice a month, as was the case for the assigned nephrologist to make necessary adjustments to the patient's treatment plan as well as checking on the patient's overall well-being.

I've heard that women make up about 77% of all healthcare professionals, but in this operation, it was 100%. Oh, I forgot there was one male who worked there. He was the guy who fixed the machines if they malfunctioned—nice guy, important job, but I never knew his name.

The technicians were incredible. With roughly eighteen patients per the three daily shifts, they typically would handle three to four patients at a time, staggering the start and finishing times like air traffic controllers. They were all pretty good at their job, but of course I had my favorites. I don't know what it's like at other facilities, but the respect, care, and kindness shown to the patients by the staff at our center is amazing.

The nurses and technicians, for the most part, are young women who began this career choice in their twenties or early thirties. One of the small things I particularly appreciated was how they all referred to the patients by their surname with the appropriate handle of Mr., Mrs., or Ms.—never getting too comfortable. They were friendly and humorous at times but always respectful. This may not seem like much, but when you're on your last leg completely vulnerable and dependent on these young people for your survival, even a modicum of respect goes a long way in the restoration of your dignity.

As I said, I had my favorites: Kisha the tech and Brandi the nurse. Techs wore these paper-thin white lab coats (if you can call them that), and nurses distinguished themselves by wearing blue-colored coats of the same material.

Brandi is a fast-walking, fast-talking bundle of energy with a heart of gold. She not only distinguished herself with her lab coat but also with her multiple hairstyle colors and footwear, especially her pink rubber boots. She was the first nurse to take care of me when I started dialysis at the center. I was confused, overwhelmed, and feeling awful on my first day—like the first day of kindergarten when your mother dropped you off at school. Her knowledge and bedside manner made me feel comfortable in what was a very uncomfortable situation for me. I felt like she took me under her wings and would not release me to anyone else until she was sure that they would do right by me. She is a natural caregiver but surprisingly fell into this profession by a twist of fate.

When she was just nineteen years old living her best life as she puts it and working at one of the big box stores, her father was diagnosed with ESRD. The youngest of her siblings, she quickly changed course and began training as a hemodialysis technician. Fast forward sixteen years, she's still in the business, working initially as a technician for eleven years before completing her associate nursing degree and becoming a nurse. She once told me, "I didn't choose this profession. This profession chose me." As of this writing, her father is still surviving on dialysis at the age of seventy-five.

Kisha's journey into health-care was, by all accounts, pure happenstance. She was at the hair salon when her stylist asked her if she would be interested in working as a dialysis technician. Apparently, one of the stylist's other clients worked at DaVita and made it known that they were looking to hire additional staff—it's amazing how much business gets done on the golf course and apparently in the hair salon.

At the time, Kisha was working as a Corrections Officer at the Maryland State Women's Prison; a criminal justice major in college, she was four years deep in her chosen field of study. Always looking for something different and to keep her busy, she accepted the challenge and applied for the job. She completed the ninety-day inculcation, which includes class work and hands-on training, and fell in love with the work. She's been a technician for nine years and, in my opinion, the best there is.

Kisha now trains the new hires but still handles patients with kindness and care. Technicians don't become certified (CCHT, Certified Clinical Hemodialysis Technician) until after they complete eighteen months of service. She tries her best to instill in her trainees not only the technical aspects of the job but also the soft skills needed to comfort the patients.

For me, Kisha made what was a stressful experience bearable with her humor, attentiveness, and overall cheerful disposition. Her attention to detail and genuine concern for each patient are remarkable, and once Brandi turned me over to the techs, I didn't want anyone other than Kisha to handle my care, although I reluctantly had to share her because she made all her patients feel the same way. I asked this married mother of two how she keeps an upbeat attitude among such daily misery and suffering. She said, "I love making people laugh and feel good. That's always been my goal since I was younger. I'm just silly, I guess."

One of the biggest financial concerns in a person's life is the cost of health insurance. Whether it be for a family or an individual, it's typically too risky to go without coverage. The cost of health insurance is only superseded by the cost of medical care without health insurance. The inability to pay healthcare debt is by far the leading cause of personal bankruptcy in the United States.

So imagine the cost associated with kidney failure: the constant visits to the nephrologist, the blood work, the medications, and the surgeries. On top of that, add dialysis treatment three times a week for the rest of your life! For example, each dialysis treatment alone costs $5,128 in 2022 and $5,487 in 2023—not including the drugs administered and other incidentals! This is three times per week, four weeks per month. My August 2022 monthly bill from my dialysis center was $86,700. Bear in mind that the median annual household income in the United States in 2022 was around $75,000. Without insurance, the affordability of long-term (even short-term) dialysis treatment is out of the question for most families.

But here's the upside to this daunting financial burden; in 1972, congress passed and President Richard M. Nixon signed (yes *that* President Nixon) the Social Security Amendments of 1972. A provision was added that extended Medicare coverage to individuals with ESRD regardless of their age. This was *huge*!

Medicare has two parts: Part A and Part B. Part A covers surgeries, in-patient hospital care, lab tests, and home health care. Part B covers doctor visits, outpatient care, medical equipment, and some preventive services. My background as a former insurance professional compels me to add some safe harbor wording here. By no means is this a comprehensive review or analysis of the coverage provided, and you must refer to the actual policy to understand the coverage specifics. Okay, enough legal (CYA) mumble jumble.

From the medicare.gov or ssa.gov/Medicare website, I learned that Medicare is the federal health insurance program for people aged sixty-five and older, under sixty-five with certain disabilities, and of any age with end-stage renal disease (ESRD) (permanent kidney failure requiring dialysis or a kidney transplant).

This declaration of disability also entitles you to prematurely collect your Social Security retirement benefits. However, one needs 40 credits of work (at least ten years) to qualify for retirement benefits—this is known as Social Security Disability Income or SSDI. The amount of your benefit is based on your highest thirty-five years of earnings. If you have fewer than thirty-five years of earnings, years without work count as zero. To keep up with inflation, benefits are adjusted at the beginning of each new year via cost-of-living adjustments.

There is also another Social Security program known as Supplemental Security Income (SSI) that requires no work credits to qualify. This was not my experience, so I won't indulge in a discussion about that.

For ESRD patients, Medicare coverage does not start until one has been on dialysis for at least three months (mine started in August of 2022) and is in force until twelve months after one stops dialysis or three years after one receives a transplant. My Social Security payments did not start for another three or four months after my Medicare coverage began.

Between Medicare and SSDI, a tremendous financial burden was lifted off my shoulders.

One of the most anticipated procedures I looked forward to was having my catheter removed. It is common practice to keep the catheter in until it is certain that your fistula is working properly before proceeding with removal of your catheter. After a few painful failed attempts, my arm was not quite ready. My fistula did not mature in the predicted four to six weeks, so I had to continue using the catheter. After four months, it was finally removed on Friday, November 18, 2022, and the use of my arm fistula began on Monday, November 21.

The Saturday before, I took the longest shower I can ever remember taking. The joy I felt was reminiscent of playing in the fire hydrant on hot summer days when I was a kid—back then, some (un) law-abiding citizens would take it upon themselves to relieve the neighborhood of the oppressive heat of the day before the firemen would come along and put an end to the party.

Around that same time, as I made my way across the parking lot on a dark morning in December heading to my dialysis treatment, I noticed that I no longer heard my foot slapping against the pavement as I stepped. I couldn't believe the miraculous change that occurred without warning. I just looked to the sky and gave thanks for this gift; I remember smiling the whole morning through my treatment. I could hardly wait to return to my old trail that weekend—as I walked that trail, I left a trail of tears praising and thanking God for this blessing.

I finally understood what my mother meant when she would blurt out now and then the words of the psalmist: "I lift up my eyes to hills; from whence cometh my help? My help comes from the Lord!"

CHAPTER 7

Getting Testy

Let me start by saying I am a patient; I am not a doctor. Like most things in life, experiences vary from person to person; this is *my* experience.

With the help of my social worker, I scheduled my appointment with Social Security and my assessments with a few transplant centers within the first month of being on dialysis. It was explained to me that it's a good idea to get on as many transplant waiting lists as possible, but the centers needed to be within two hours of travel time (or inside of 250 nautical miles) in case I received a call letting me know that a matching kidney was available. Deceased donor kidneys can only be preserved for twenty-four to forty-eight hours, so time is of the essence.

Fewer than one in seven end-stage kidney disease patients make the deceased donor waitlist. My assessments were scheduled with three transplant centers: The University of Maryland, Johns Hopkins (both approximately thirteen miles from my home), and Georgetown University Hospital, about thirty-six miles away. The University of Virginia (136 miles down the road) was on standby just in case.

On June 8, I was informed via email that I was scheduled for a telemedicine appointment at the University of Maryland Transplant Center on Tuesday, June 28, at 8:00 a.m. That was a relatively quick response considering I had only been on dialysis a month—I told you that Chekana was the real deal.

To prepare for the appointment, I needed to answer the following questions at least forty-eight hours before the appointment, or the appointment would be canceled. Cancelled? There was no way I was going to blow this opportunity. My thought was, *Let's hurry up, and get this two-to-five-year waiting period started!*

They needed to know my weight and height and if I am or ever was a smoker or user of alcohol or drugs. They also needed a list of my current medications, medical histories, and previous surgeries. But wait, that's not all. I needed to provide them with information on any family members with health issues and if they were still alive or deceased.

On June 28, I had the telemedicine visit—COVID-19 was still in effect, so this is how things were done at the time. This was a well-coordinated call that lasted about two and a half to three hours. I spoke with a nephrologist, an anesthesiologist, a surgeon, a psychologist, a couple of nurses, and I can't remember who else, but it was a very informative and hope-filled call.

In general, before anyone can be listed as a kidney transplant candidate, they must go through an evaluation process as determined by the transplant center. Typically, the evaluation includes the prospect's medical history as mentioned above and a host of other tests as listed below:

- Physical exam (BMI typically 40 or less)
- Psychological exam (if on meds are you compliant)
- Blood test to check your liver, heart, and immune system and screen for certain diseases, especially cancer
- Chest X-ray
- Antibody test
- Blood and tissue typing tests to determine which type of kidney donor you are most compatible
- Kidney function test (must be $\leq$20% to be evaluated)

- Dental exam
- Nutrition evaluation
- Cardiopulmonary tests, including an electrocardiogram (EKG), cardiac stress test, and pulmonary function test to be sure of your body's ability to sustain the strenuous surgery
- Imaging tests, including CT scans, abdominal ultrasound, renal ultrasound, and vascular ultrasound
- Other tests as deemed necessary by the transplant center

There is no upper age limit for a kidney transplant. It all depends on how healthy you are—in fact, most transplant recipients are fifty or older. I've heard anecdotes of people in their eighties and nineties receiving transplants. But to have a serious chance of being accepted, they must be in very good health otherwise.

I was approved and listed on their deceased donor waitlist in August—yippee!

Test tubes were sent to my home monthly, and blood was drawn at the dialysis center and sent via overnight mail to the transplant center. I assume it was blood and tissue typing test, but I can't say for certain. I just knew it was required to remain on the list.

I had applied to Johns Hopkins and Georgetown around the same time I contacted the University of Maryland but heard nothing for months—let me correct that: I did receive a call from a scheduling coordinator (for lack of a better title) from Johns Hopkins in June or July informing me that they were backed up and I would hear from someone in October. That was better than the response I received from Georgetown. That person told me that they weren't scheduling evaluations for anyone who had been on dialysis for less than three months—the woman later denied she said that, but I know what I heard; after all, this was extremely important to me.

In early October, I received a call from the Johns Hopkins Kidney Transplant Coordinator informing me that my evaluation appointment was scheduled for October 13, 2022, at 2:20 p.m. Her name was Billie, and although she had been a nurse since 2016, she was new to Hopkins Transplant Center, starting there permanently in April of 2022.

This was another well-coordinated telemedicine visit, although it did not take as long because there was lots of pre-call literature and forms to sign as well as an informative video fully explaining the transplantation process. In addition, a thirty-minute conference call was scheduled with the Johns Hopkins social worker for Tuesday, October 25, 2022, at 12:30 p.m. I needed to have my support team on the call as well. I invited my two children, and they agreed to participate.

The official purpose of the call with the social worker was to inform me about the challenges that lie ahead regarding cost, insurance coverage, needed caretaker support, post-op limitations, medication requirements, waiting time on the deceased donor list, need to be ready at the drop of a hat in the event I received a call that a kidney was available, etc. The unofficial purpose was to scare the crap out of me and my children!

To my total surprise, at the end of the call, my son asked the social worker if he could be tested to see if he was a match. He was only thirty-one years old. My heart sank! I was so taken by this gesture of generosity that I didn't know whether to laugh or cry, so I did both at the same time.

It didn't matter to me if he was a match or not, just the pure fact that he wanted to be tested was enough for me. You know you raise your children to be the best version of themselves and a better version of you. Out of love, there are so many sacrifices made for them throughout the years that their well-being becomes who you are, your identity. But love is not always reciprocated—at least not the action kind. To know that your child appreciates you, wants to alleviate your burden and needs and wants you to continue living, it's too much. I can hardly write this part of my story without being overcome with emotion. To this day, I don't know if my son truly understands what he did for me.

I received a letter in the mail from Billie dated November 1, 2022, informing me of the required next steps to expedite the workup process and tests that needed to be completed in the next sixty days for my case to be presented to the medical review team.

The requirements were pretty much the same as they were for the University of Maryland with a few exceptions.

- Lab work was to be conducted at Hopkins or could be ordered by my PCP.
- Diagnostic testing:
    - Dobutamine stress echo to rule out inducible ischemia; for the results to be acceptable, I needed to achieve a MTHR of 85%
    - Colonoscopy if not done in the past 5 or 10 years
- Consultations:
    - Letter of dental health clearance
    - Kidney biopsy report
- Others: immunization record; hepatitis B vaccination documentation

The letter went on to state that if I had completed any of these tests in the last twelve months to please make a request to have them faxed to their office. "What? Who still uses faxes?" I said. The letter further went on to say incomplete testing will not be accepted blah, blah, blah, yada yada yada.

When am I supposed to get all this done? I only have two good days a week and scheduling doctor's appointments isn't exactly an on-demand endeavor. Ugh! This is so frustrating!

I called my PCP to see what he could do, and he advised that it would be better to have Hopkins schedule the appointments. *Et Tu, Brute?* I was feeling like I was being abandoned with a boat load of things to be accomplished in a short period of time.

On top of that, in September of that same year, I had a telemedicine visit with a pulmonologist to have a sleep study assessment. It had been brought to my attention that I snore while sleeping—but it's worth noting that I never snore when sleeping alone. Hmm? In all seriousness, people with chronic kidney disease often experience sleep apnea.

On October 12, I spent the night at GBMC's sleep center and was found to have severe sleep apnea. I was referred to the Johns Hopkins Pharmaquip facility where I was equipped with a continuous positive airway pressure machine—I began using my CPAP machine in December. I had to remind myself not to panic. "Que Sera, Sera (whatever will be, will be)." It's hard by the yard but a cinch by the inch.

Billie and I worked out our testing scheduling issues, not necessarily in the suggested sixty days but close enough to keep me in the queue. The tests that were not yet completed had been scheduled, so I thought.

Meanwhile, my son informed me the first week of January that his transplant donor coordinator can't send him the order for his labs because I had not completed all my testing yet. I was hot! I asked my son for his coordinator's phone number so that we can have a conference call and get the ball rolling. When we had the call, his coordinator was reluctant to give me any information because of privacy laws and their protocols and procedures. I said to her impatiently, "This is my son. There's no secret here. I know who my donor is, and he knows who his recipient is!" She kept repeating herself and referred me back to my coordinator.

Why can't we just have one coordinator and cut through some of this red tape? I was so upset, and I hung up the phone while she was saying goodbye. I started to feel like I was getting the runaround, so I called Billie to see what was what. I needed to ask her if she was in constant communication with the donor coordinating transplant nurse and why aren't they one and the same?

Billie's a very busy lady, so of course, I got her voicemail. This too was frustrating in the beginning and to be honest all the way through, until I learned after the fact just how busy Billie was. She wasn't just my coordinating nurse; she is juggling close to two hundred patients in varying stages of the process all at one time. A typical workday for her consists of reviewing patient's charts, speaking to patients, returning emails, preparing for clinic, preparing reports for the selection committee, and requesting testing from patient's doctors, just to name a few.

When Billie and I did speak, she was very patient with me and acknowledged my frustration. I asked about the coordinator issue, and she explained the importance of separation of church and state so to speak. They want to be sure the donor is doing this of their own free will and that this is purely altruistic and not by coercion or incentivized by monetary gain. She added that she would do what she could to forward my completed results to the donor coordinating nurse to see if we could at least start the blood testing process with my son.

I also asked her if she could give me the three to five major reasons why someone would not qualify to be a recipient of a kidney transplant and the same for someone not qualifying to become a donor. Her response was if either had active cancer, advanced cardiovascular disease, active drug use, or uncontrolled mental health issues, neither would qualify. I was confident that we would pass those tests. I hope!

Billie and I have sort of special bond because I was her first patient and this was my first transplant. She had a rather circuitous route in becoming a nurse. Coming out of high school, she thought she wanted to be a teacher but instead became a young mother and put her formal education on hold for a while. Then she became a hairstylist and then a real estate agent before her then-seventeen-year-old son convinced her to resume her education and begin college with him. So she went back to school for nursing and graduated in 2016. It's amazing how we first try to inspire our children, and they end up inspiring us.

Fast forward to 2020, she became a travel nurse during the pandemic, and the kidney transplant job was actually one of her last travel assignments. The assignment was for thirteen weeks, and she loved it so much that she wanted to stay (and they wanted her to stay too), but they did not have any openings at the time, so she left and took a job at another hospital, which she did not like. As fate would have it, a couple of months into that job, Hopkins called her and asked her to return, and she's been there ever since.

What I find interesting about Billie's journey is that both her mother and grandmother were nurses. Why was she trying to be something other than what is naturally in her bloodline? I guess we can all be guilty of that on our way to finding our destiny. Sometimes, we run all over the place looking for what's right in front of us—you can run, but you can't hide; nature has the final word, or as my mother used to say, "What's at the bottom of the well eventually comes up in the bucket."

CHAPTER 8

Wait and Believe

Let me start by saying I am a patient; I am not a doctor. Like most things in life, experiences vary from person to person; this is *my* experience.

When I think of God, I think of the unknown. In other words, God is the creator of everything I know and the keeper of everything I don't know. So when I don't have knowledge or understanding of something, I take it to God. When I have no idea what, how, where, or when something happened or will happen, I ask for wisdom and understanding, and then I wait, believing if it is for me to know, it will be revealed to me.

I did not know why I was dealt this hand at this point in my life. But you know what, at this stage of my disease and treatment, it didn't really matter. I just know that I am here and it must be for my edification, so there is no need to worry. Fate has been too good to me to start questioning it now. The book of James in the Bible expresses it better than I can:

> Count it all joy, my brothers, when you meet trials of various kinds, for you know that the testing of your faith produces steadfastness. And let steadfastness have its full effect, that you may be perfect and complete, lacking in nothing. If any of you lacks wisdom, let him ask God, who gives generously to all without reproach, and it will be given him. <u>But let</u>

> him ask in faith, with no doubting, for the one who doubts is like a wave of the sea that is driven and tossed by the wind. For that person must not suppose that he will receive anything from the Lord; he is a double-minded man, unstable in all his ways. (James 1:2–8)

I am committed to seeing this thing through and if it be God's will that I receive a deceased donor kidney, I am willing to wait as long as it takes. At this point, I had been on dialysis for about six months—six months down, maybe another twenty-four to forty-eight more to go. I had my routine down pat, and I had done all that I needed to do in preparation of receiving that call.

I did not miss any dialysis treatments. I diligently followed the kidney diet and received all smiley faces on my reports from Sue, the dietician every time—I thought this was corny at first, but I started to anxiously await my report card. It served as confirmation that I was doing everything right and motivated me to stay on the path.

I lowered my sugar intake (of course), put a halt to the salt, and avoided foods high in potassium and phosphorous (read food labels—you'd be surprised) including some fruits and vegetables. It's pretty intuitive that excess sodium and sugar are not good for your health, but not so much for potassium and phosphorus. But as a kidney patient with limited nutrient balancing abilities, I also had to do what was necessary to limit these nutrients because unhealthy levels can wreak havoc on the heart and bones. I was prescribed Auryxia to help control my phosphorous level and to treat my anemia—I took two tablets with each meal.

I put my finances in order, made all of my doctor appointments, completed my surgeries (catheter inserted and removed, fistula in place and working), completed my Medicare and SSDI paperwork, and had my support team in place. I just needed to keep my mind right. No negativity in my sphere—feed the faith, and starve the doubt. Shout-out to "Marvelous" Marvin Hagler, may he rest in peace.

It is truly a blessing to qualify and ultimately receive a kidney transplant under any circumstance. Finding a match can be a long and arduous process. As mentioned in a previous chapter, just qualifying to be on the waitlist can be challenging, and there is no guarantee that you will remain on the list until you receive a matching kidney—health conditions can change over time.

On any given day, there are over 90,000 patients on the deceased donor waitlist in the United States. Per the Organ Procurement Transplant Network (OPTN), on average, patients are on the wait list three to five years. These numbers are for adults only—meaning aged eighteen or older. There is a prioritization system in place with regard to how deceased donor kidneys are allocated.

Blood type and organ size weigh into the allocation of every donated organ, but specific to deceased kidney donor transplants, the following additions are taken into consideration:

1. If you were a prior living donor
2. Your time on the wait list
3. The availability of your specific blood type
4. Compatibility of donor and recipient immune systems
5. Your overall health condition
6. Your distance from the donor hospital
7. Your age
8. Your willingness to accept a lower-grade donation

With my headphones on, eyes closed most of the time even while awake, I listened and believed that whatever happened, I was going to be all right. I love most types of music, from classical to blues, jazz to country, soul to easy listening, and, yes, even some rap and rock 'n' roll. But when it comes down to focusing my spirit on higher things, there's nothing like good old gospel music for me. So on my dialysis mornings, I primarily listened to music, audiobooks, sermons, and Earl Nightingale's oration on *The Strangest Secret*—spoiler alert: "We become what we think about."

However, for reasons unknown to me, once the new year began, I almost exclusively listened to the gospel playlists I had created. There were days when water would involuntarily fall from my eyes. The techs would ask me, "Are you okay, Mr. Macoy? Is everything all right?"

I would reply with a trembling voice as the tears rolled down my face, "Absolutely everything is all right, just overwhelmed with joy. Would you be so kind and hand me a paper towel?"

Around this time, some of the people who were with me at the early part of my diagnosis and treatment started to fade away—disappointing yes but not shockingly surprising. Early in my career, I used to ride a commuter train, and I realized then that everyone who gets on the train with you doesn't necessarily get off at the same stop. The good news is this: usually at the same time someone is exiting others are getting on board.

True love never dies—and the other kind is not worth worrying about. Sometimes, the thought of losing a loved one is just too much to bear, and although the physical pain is with the sick, their loved ones have their own emotional pain to cope with. But I remain hopeful. In the poetic words of the singer-songwriter Michael Franks, "Someday, when all our hearts are reassembled, love will reconnect us once again. And we'll resume our time together."

I learned a neat trick while going through this particular crisis; if you want someone out of your life, just tell them how much you need them. It takes effort to bring down a tree, but leaves come and go—rooted trees stand tall, while leaves, well, leave.

I've always been amazed at how many people are quick to offer their thoughts and prayers when they hear about another's sorrow or suffering, but little else. Plenty are willing to come to your funeral but won't come to your aid in your time of need. Maybe, just maybe, if as many people had come to your aid as those willing to pay their respects, you may have lived a little longer.

But it's not wise to condemn people for not knowing what they don't know. The wise thing to do in my opinion is to find the meaning in your suffering. Suffering wasn't made just for some. If you live long enough, you come to the realization that anything can happen to anybody. You begin to understand that no matter who you are or how important you think you are, days are only given out one at a time.

Over the years, my brother and I would often laugh about how people comment on another person's success or failure. They'll often say, "I always knew" that he or she would end up like this or that, regardless of the outcome, win or lose, succeed or fail; they always knew. There's something in human nature that makes us want to be right when in actuality we're only right on average about thirty percent of the time. Our unwillingness to admit that there is a certain randomness to life is just too frightening to accept—so we rationalize.

CHAPTER 9

I Struck a Match

Let me start by saying I am a patient; I am not a doctor. Like most things in life, experiences vary from person to person; this is *my* experience.

As time passed on, I continued to wait, hoping that my son's testing was progressing and believing against all odds that a deceased matching kidney might show up at the front end rather than the back end of the average wait time. If one is fortunate enough to receive a kidney from a living donor, there are clearly some advantages. But when you're on dialysis and interested in getting off dialysis like I was, any kidney donation would suffice.

I learned from my transplant coordinating nurse (Billie) that donated kidneys are ranked or classified. That each donor kidney is given a score of 0 to 100, based on things like age, ethnicity, cause of death, chronic diseases at time of death, and drug use. I'm sure there are other considerations, but this is what I remember. For example, a Kidney Donor Profile Index or KDPI of 10 means there's a probability that the kidney will last 90% longer than all other donated kidneys, and a score of 90 means it will last only 10% longer.

I remember signing a consent form expressing my willingness to accept a deceased kidney donor with hepatitis C if one became available. This of course would be a lower classified kidney and most people would take a pass, but by accepting it, I would improve my odds of receiving a kidney faster—besides, there was now a cure for hep C. This was how determined I was to get off dialysis.

Optimally, a living donor is preferred. There is less wait time, there's the possibly of avoiding dialysis altogether, and there's the ability to plan ahead. Oh yeah, and on average, living donor transplants last longer than those from a deceased donor. But even with that, over 50% of willing living donors don't qualify for various testing and health reasons. Imagine having someone willing to make that lifesaving sacrifice for you only to be told they don't meet the standards—how demoralizing!

But in the event your living donor's tissue or blood type does not match yours but otherwise qualifies to be a donor, there are programs available whereby your donor could swap their matching kidney with another family or transplant patient that matches with your tissue and blood type. This is an ingenious way of keeping hope alive when the direct donor's blood or tissue typing does not match their targeted recipient. It's been reported that one kidney donation can affect eight different people with this crossmatching method.

However, certain criteria need to be met before becoming a living donor:

- You must be over the age of eighteen.
- You must be willing to commit to the pre-donation evaluation process, surgery, and the burden of recovery.
- You must be in good health and psychological condition.
- You must have a compatible blood type (not necessarily so if swapping).
- You must have compatible crossmatch—you are not compatible based on antibodies (not necessarily so if swapping).
- You must have normal kidney function.

In certain situations, you must meet additional requirements to become a living donor. For example, if your body mass index (BMI) is greater than 30, you have high blood pressure or a history of kidney stones.

You cannot be a living donor if you:

- are under the of age eighteen;
- have heart disease, diabetes, or cancer;
- have chronic kidney problems; and
- have any conditions that may jeopardize your health by kidney donation (e.g., pregnancy, being underweight, etc.).

On January 18, 2023, I received a text from my son advising me that he completed his blood work and urinalysis. On the 19th, he sent me the results. His blood was O+, and I replied, "You've got that universal blood—awesome!" The irony in this is that people with blood type O can donate or give blood to anyone but can only receive blood or an organ donation from other people with blood type O and thus tend to be on the wait list longer than people with A or AB blood types.

The DaVita nephrologist had got wind of the fact that my son was being tested to see if he was a match for me. She was very pleased and gave me the stats on the survival rate for living donor recipients versus deceased donor recipients. The number I remember her sharing with me was twice as long—like twenty years versus ten years on average.

Whenever she made her bimonthly visits to the DaVita center, she would ask for updates about my son and the testing progress. I shared some of my frustrations with her about the process but let her know that we were still on track.

Later that month, my son and I talked about his EGFR, and I didn't like the number I saw. I had some literature indicating that donors permanently lose 20–25% of their kidney function and were at risk of developing hypertension. I said, "I appreciate the offer, son, but I don't want that for you. I'll just continue to wait on the deceased donor list. It'll be all right." Unlike with living donors, there is no age limit on deceased kidney donations. I met a guy who received a kidney from a six-year-old girl when he was fifty-six, and twelve years later, he was still going strong.

But my son said, "Let's just wait and see before you make any final decisions. I think I can clean up my lifestyle and maintain going forward." He had been taking a protein supplement and had not been drinking enough water.

I informed the nephrologist of the latest development and let her know that I would just wait for a deceased donor kidney. She kept expressing that people who donate a kidney go on to live full and healthy lives and if the surgery team thought that there was any concern with my son's donation, they would not proceed. I listened to what she had to say, but in my mind, it didn't matter what she said. I just knew I wasn't going to put my son in jeopardy.

A couple of weeks later, my son called me and said things had improved. He indeed cleaned up his act and was given the actual GFR test instead of the EGFR and the numbers were high enough where I was comfortable with continuing on with the process. On March 3, he informed me that his in-person appointment with Johns Hopkins was scheduled for Monday, March 13 at 7:00 a.m. This would be an all-day event where he would complete his final fitness test including psych evaluation, blood work, urinalysis, EKG, and chest X-ray as well as meet with his surgeon and nurses. Five months after finding out that my son was willing to be tested, the back and forth, the uncertainty—this was really happening!

The sacrifice, steadfastness, and discipline required by my son as he navigated through this mental, emotional, and physical gauntlet dwarfed anything I experienced personally. Despite the hurdles put before him, some intentional, some inadvertently, he remained committed to the process. He never wavered.

This speaks volumes about his character. He never talks about it and never toots his own horn or expects any special celebration or recognition. My son epitomizes the late basketball coach John Wooden's quote regarding character: "Be more concerned with your character than your reputation, because your character is what you are, while your reputation is merely what others think you are."

When he was growing up, I would often talk to him about just doing what needs to be done without looking for accolades from outsiders—to just try to be good for goodness sake. I'd Socratically ask, "Do you want to be this kind of guy or that kind of guy? Choose wisely, and then be him!"

I asked if he wanted me to make flight arrangements for his visit to Baltimore, but he declined because he was bringing his dog with him. He arrived in town that Sunday evening before his appointment. I wanted to go along with him but could not due to my 6:45 a.m. standing appointment with dialysis. It was a long day for the both of us. I was taking my normal midday nap when he returned, and when I awoke, he was asleep. We had a brief chance to catch up on Tuesday before he was back on the road that afternoon arriving home around midnight—ah to be young.

Because kidney failure occurs four times as much in Black Americans when compared to their White counterparts, an APOL 1 risk variant test is given to be sure the donor is not at an increased risk of developing kidney disease down the line.

The APOL 1 gene plays a role in immunity. This gene evolved over time (thousands of years) in African people to fight against a specific parasite that caused African sleeping sickness. It was a good thing in its proper setting, but for those African descendants in the diaspora, it has been known to cause a higher risk for kidney disease if a person has two of these mutated gene variants. Bottom line, if you have two of these mutated genes variants (one from father, one from mother), you are at a higher risk of developing chronic kidney disease.

Approximately 13% of Black Americans have two APOL 1 kidney risk variants compared to 0.1% for other races. My son did not have two and therefore was not at a higher risk. On March 23, he sent me a text that said, "It's done!" He had been cleared!

He had completed everything he needed to do and passed with flying colors. All that remained was for me to complete the few items left on my checklist. This journey was almost over, I could see the light at the end of the tunnel, and it wasn't a train headed my way. My son and I had a discussion once about being a little nervous now that we were so close to the finish line—not about the potential surgery but about coming this far and some fluke coming out of nowhere derailing the whole thing. We talked about being overly cautious during this waiting period and decided not to worry because if this miracle was meant to happen, it would; besides, we had beaten so many odds already, it seemed destined to happen. However, in the meantime, we agreed that we would not do anything to tempt fate—even unknowingly contracting COVID could delay or disrupt the progress.

As mentioned before, so many concerned loved ones had gone down this path only to be rejected at the last minute for one reason or another. I was surprised to hear that it's not unusual for individuals to profess a desire to be tested as a possible donor, only to never follow through with getting tested. What a cruel game to play on the emotions of a desperate patient. This was sad to me when I heard about that; I'm not often surprised by the callousness of people, but this revelation caught me flat-footed. On the other hand, this information made me respect my son even more.

My son, my son—my son was born on a Saturday, in fact, the Saturday before Father's Day. Like my daughter, he was born the day before a day designated for me, again, another sign that my child was supposed to come before me. I prayed for a son and made a sacred promise to God Almighty that if He answered my prayer, well, that's between God and me.

I remember the time leading up to his birth and being fascinated with a tune by John Coltrane's quartet titled, <u>The Promise (Live at Birdland)</u>. In particular, the solo by pianist McCoy Tyner enthralled me. I must have played that song three or four times a day from the time my son was just a twinkle in my eye to the day he was born. There was something about the song's slow crescendo that was mesmerizing.

The tune starts with a calm Coltrane saxophone solo as the rhythm section keeps tempo in the background, and just when Coltrane is about to take us down a wandering road as he is known to do, McCoy's piano solo steps in to keep things mellow before taking us on his own melodic roller-coaster ride of twist and turns. This solo takes up the middle of the piece before he brings us back down and allows Coltrane's saxophone to once again take the lead. He, in my opinion, has now set the tone for Coltrane to take us on his own melodic world wind of sound that crescendos at a less chaotic and esoteric pace before everything comes back together by the song's end.

So when the nurse came to me as I sat in the waiting room (no delivery room for me) around noon informing me that I was the proud father of a healthy baby boy, I knew what I would call him—the promise! This is who this baby was, and this is the man this boy would become.

I used to refer to my son as a physical genius because he could do all sorts of physical things well before you'd expect a child of his age—little did I know.

CHAPTER 10

Transplantation

Let me start by saying I am a patient; I am not a doctor. Like most things in life, experiences vary from person to person; this is *my* experience.

The first successful kidney transplant surgery was done in 1954. It involved identical twin brothers Ronald (donor) and Richard (recipient) Herrick. They were twenty-three years old when the operation took place. Richard was dying from chronic nephritis. A side note: my daughter taught me, when she was a first-year medical student, that in medicine, the suffix *itis* means "inflammation or infection."

This was very controversial at the time and posed ethical dilemmas, both spiritual and medical. Healthy people were not supposed to be operated on—remember the Hippocratic Oath: "First do no harm." But after numerous tests, discussions, and warnings, the family agreed to proceed. There was no guarantee that this would work. As a matter of fact, the first successful allotransplantation (meaning same species, e.g., human to human) was attempted in Paris a year earlier. The kidney of a mother killed in an auto accident was donated to her sixteen-year-old son but was rejected after only twenty-two days.

But the doctors reasoned that because the brothers were identical twins, meaning they shared the exact same genetic makeup, Richard's immune system would not identify his brother's kidney as foreign and therefore would not attack it. It worked! Richard went on to marry one of the operating room nurses, and they ended up having two children before Richard succumbed to another kidney-related problem and died in 1963. His brother, Ronald, went on to live to the ripe old age of seventy-nine, leaving this earth in 2010 but leaving behind a road map and legacy that have extended the lives of so many.

As a matter of fact, according to OPTN, there were a total of 27,332 kidney transplants in the year 2023 alone, of which 26,543 were adults—with 6,290 donated kidneys coming from living donors. Kidney transplant advancement has come a long way since the early days. Initially only done with identical twins, then fraternal twins, and then siblings; and it wasn't until 1962 that the first successful deceased donor kidney transplant was completed.

Present-day adult kidney transplants received by age range were as follows:

1. Age 50–64 represented 39%.
2. Age 65 and older at 25%.
3. Age 35–49 at 23%.
4. Eighteen- to thirty-four-year-olds were 10% of the adult recipients.

So as you can see, kidney failure can occur at any age. One strange fact I discovered was that upward to 18% of deceased kidney donations come from individuals who died from a drug overdose. That was shocking to me at first. But the more I thought about it, the more it made sense, considering a majority of drug overdoses occur in otherwise healthy young people. Thank goodness they were at least cognizant enough to sign the necessary paperwork or driver's license to consent to organ donation at some point during their life.

I want to underscore this point: <u>every year, there are over 90,000 people on the wait list for a kidney transplant, and a</u>

<u>new person is added to the transplant network every ten minutes.</u> It's been widely reported that fourteen people die every day waiting on the wait list for a kidney.

It can be an arduous process even with a willing living donor. As mentioned before, over 50% of living candidates willing to make this gracious sacrifice don't qualify for one reason or another.

But despite its challenges, the kidney community has made great strides over the years. Today, even altruistic living donations are on the rise from people with no relation or personal connection to the recipient, just a willingness to reduce another's suffering.

With a better understanding of the immune system and the development of more effective immunosuppressant drugs, the medical community continues to improve and extend the functionality rates of donated kidneys. Couple that with further research, medical advances, technological improvements in surgical procedures, and living donor participation, the future looks very bright for transplant patients. In fact, there are early discussions taking place presently regarding xenotransplantation (cross species) with some of the same ethical and medical dilemmas discussed in 1954 regarding the Herrick twins allograft.

I received a call from the transplant nurse (Kathy) in March, to schedule an appointment with the transplant surgeon on April 5, 2023. I had been cleared medically and financially to be listed on the kidney transplant list. The appointment time was 11:30 a.m., forty-five minutes after completion of my morning dialysis treatment. I didn't mind the forty-minute drive because I was so close to the finish line.

Of course, there was one more hurdle. "Billie, what now?" I needed to have the dental clearance form completed by my dentist before she could present my case to the selection committee.

You have got to be kidding me! Fortunately, I had scheduled a dental appointment a month earlier and was able to get that done the day before I met with the surgeon.

This seemed to be a moot point, as I had already received a letter from the surgical director dated April 3 notifying me that I had been listed as Active (Status 1) on the United Network for Organ Sharing (UNOS) with Hopkins. UNOS is the nonprofit corporation that operates OPTN. I had already been listed back in August of 2022 by The University of Maryland, and by this point, I also had an approved living donor. I guess wires were crossed, and they were just making sure *all* the *I*s were dotted and *all* the *T*s were crossed.

Dr. D was my surgeon. His official title was Surgical Director, Kidney Transplantation. This guy has mastered the rhetorical triangle of ethos, pathos, and logos. He was great, the kind of doctor that exudes so much confidence that he makes you feel confident. He was around my age, maybe three or four years younger, and had been in his current position close to fourteen years. He told me that I was a great candidate for transplant and that he did not foresee any problems with the surgery. He explained the procedure and showed me the scan of my abdomen and how and where the new kidney would be placed in my body. He spent plenty of time with me and answered all of my questions.

I asked if he was going to remove my old kidneys. His response was, "No," and explained why. I asked why the new kidney was being placed in my lower-right abdomen instead of my back, and he explained why. I asked how long the surgery would take, and he answered, "Four maybe five hours," and explained why. I asked if my son and I would be in the same operating room, and he answered, "No," and explained why. He explained the cleaning and prepping process of the donated kidney and the time allotted between removal of my son's kidney and the insertion into my body. I asked how soon we can get this done. He explained the scheduling process and advised that Kathy would notify me of the next available date. I felt good leaving that meeting and reported to dialysis the next morning feeling confident about my upcoming surgery.

On April 14, Kathy called again informing me that my transplant surgery had been scheduled for Thursday, May 4—hallelujah! *May the Fourth be with us!* I shared this news with my dialysis nurse Brandi and asked her to keep a tight lip; this would be our secret. I didn't want my rowboat family or any of the DaVita staff to know—sort of a survivor's remorse feeling perhaps.

I had my pre-op appointment the morning of April 18 to check my vitals and have blood work done, which took about an hour. On the 26th, a blood kit was shipped to my home with the necessary test tubes to have blood drawn at dialysis and express mailed back to Hopkins the same day. Then on May 2, I needed to drive back to Hopkins to have a COVID-19 test, as COVID testing was required for my son and me within forty-eight to seventy-two hours of surgery. If either of us tested positive, the surgery would be postponed, and finally, I needed to have my regularly scheduled dialysis treatment on Wednesday—the day before my surgery.

Day of surgery

We arrived at the hospital at six thirty that morning. My son's surgery would take place at 10:00 a.m.—last chance to back out! He was cool as a cucumber, at least that's the way he appeared on the outside. My sister flew in town the day before and was there to check us both into the hospital—she really came through for the both of us! The three of us sat there quietly as my sister attempted to make conversation to calm her nerves.

Once my son was called back to prep for his surgery, my sister and I sat there waiting, hoping, and praying that all would go well. The donor surgery is a laparoscopic procedure (meaning minimally invasive) that requires four pinhole insertions via a telescopic rod lens system in the abdomen and a small three-inch incision just below the naval to pull the kidney out of the body. About two-and-a-half hours later, the surgeon came out and said that the surgery went very well and that my son was in recovery. *Whew! Praise the Lord!*

I was taken back to the prepping area around 1:00 or 1:30 p.m. My son was just starting to wake up around 2:00 p.m. I needed to see him and needed to lay eyes on him before my surgery, which was scheduled for around 3:00 p.m. I walked around to the other side of the hospital floor to see how he was doing. Although drowsy, he was in good spirits and jokingly wagged his index finger at me saying, "No, Mutombo,"

I said, "What?"

He said, "No rejection of my kidney," an old basketball reference—I knew then that he was all right.

Now that his kidney was out of his body and on ice being prepped to be put into my body and he was doing well and in good spirits, I had no worries. I returned to my room in preparation to be taken into the operating room. I remember being wheeled through the hallway by the anesthesiologist and entering the OR at 3:18 p.m. There was a team of nurses and doctors ready to do what they do. I greeted them all by saying, "Hello, good afternoon. It's 3:18 p.m. That's my birthday." The next thing I remember was waking up in recovery around nine o'clock(ish) and the surgeon telling me that everything went well.

The surgery lasted about four-and-a-half hours and entailed a hands-on precision technique. This wasn't a laparoscopic procedure; this required an incision, proper placement of my new kidney, connecting and sewing blood vessels, the attachment of a stent and catheter, and inserting a Jackson-Pratt closed suction system, better known as a JP drain in my abdomen. And then there's the closing of the wound—mine was closed using twenty-seven staples.

The surgery was a success! My new kidney (which I refer to as our kidney) began working immediately as far as I know. What I do know for certain is that while I lay in my hospital bed that night, the bag connected to my catheter was filling up with urine. This meant our kidney was doing its job of filtering and balancing my body fluids, and that's a great thing!

My sister was a tremendous help and stayed in my room with me and kept an eye on my son, whose room was on the other side of the floor, until she had to catch a flight back home that weekend. She was relieved by my brother who flew in from Georgia that Saturday. He was also a huge help and was there to discharge me from the hospital the following Monday and served as my driver and nurse maid for the first week of my stay at home. My sister, who was extremely generous with her time, returned the following week to pick up where he left off and watched over me the entire second week. And remember my old buddy from Los Angeles? He graciously came to be with me for two weeks after my sister returned home—the first four weeks were behind me, and I was doing better than expected!

My son only stayed in the hospital for two nights! Although sore, he checked himself out, retrieved his dog from the kennel, and rested at my home with his aunt and uncle that weekend, watching over him just to be safe. He needed to stick around for his post-surgery follow-up visit exactly one week later, and the two of us recuperated at home upon my return. Once that was over and everything checked out fine, he and his faithful companion (his dog Remington) hopped in his SUV and drove the eight hours back to North Carolina—amazing! He was advised to refrain from heavy lifting the first month or so, but there were no dietary or physical restrictions going forward—just a healthy diet routine.

I recall those prophetic words of my college professor: "Maintenance is cheaper than repair." The cost associated with our transplant surgeries from May 2 to May 8 was $116,545. This included my four-day hospital stay and the $60,000 for my son's donor operation and hospital stay but does not include any pre- and posttransplant discharge charges. All expenses associated with my son's surgery and testing were paid for by my insurance, Medicare parts A and B. In other words, there is zero out-of-pocket expense for the donor as it relates to the surgery.

It's important to remember that transplant surgery is an amazing thing and restores a lot of function and freedom to the recipient's life, but it is not a cure. It is a treatment, and therefore a regiment must be followed to maintain the health of your transplanted kidney.

CHAPTER 11

Another Beginning

Let me start by saying I am a patient; I am not a doctor. Like most things in life, experiences vary from person to person; this is *my* experience.

The day before my transplant surgery, my EGFR was 7%, and my creatinine level was 7.8. Keep in mind, the normal range for creatinine is .76–1.27. When I started dialysis almost exactly one year prior, my numbers were just about the same—stage 5 and barely holding on to any kidney function. On the day I was discharged from the hospital (four days after my surgery), my creatinine was 1.6, and my EGFR was 49%—a sevenfold improvement in just four days! Oh yeah, this was working and working well!

I didn't realize how sick I was until I got well. Although I was very active only three or four months before my official diagnosis, my kidney function had not been this efficient in three years, maybe more. Like the lifting of fog on a warm morning following a cool rainy night, my brain fog dissipated, and the clarity of my thoughts seemed to return almost immediately.

I was surprised by how little pain I felt after the surgery—and no, it wasn't the painkillers. As a matter of fact, both my son and I declined the pain meds offered to us. I was encouraged to drink plenty of water, which was a challenge considering I had grown used to consuming no more than thirty-two ounces of fluid per day over the past year. The first day following my surgery, I was able to sit up in my hospital bed, and later that day or early the next morning, I was able to sit in the chair in my room. I was also able to use the bathroom the day after my surgery, which was greeted with shock and awe by the doctors and nurses as this was yet another sign that my recovery was progressing quickly. It's recommended that the patient move around to avoid clotting, and by Sunday, I was taking laps around the hospital floor, slowly and gingerly but surely. The JP drain, which hung about six to eight inches outside of my body, made walking with tempo a struggle especially in a hospital gown.

During one of my walks, I remember seeing on a hallway bulletin board a list of how many transplants were completed by the Hopkins transplant team per month and year.

Transplants	Last Month	Last Year
Kidney	17	236
Liver	7	121
Pancreas and Kidney/Pancreas	1	4

This wasn't their first rodeo. These guys are doing on average close to twenty kidney transplants per month. According to OPTN, there were a total of 46,629 organ transplants from both deceased and living donors in 2023—approximately 60% of which were kidney transplants. The vast majority of transplants are from the organs of deceased donors, but there is an upward trend in both deceased and living donor organs. My hope is that this trend continues in a positive direction as more people realize the benefits of this lifesaving gift.

I'm sure my immunosuppressant drugs were started shortly after my surgery and continued to be administered intravenously while I was in the hospital. My final morning in the hospital was a busy one. My IV and catheter were removed, I was given a list of pharmaceuticals I needed to take and collect from the pharmacy on the way out, and I was visited by a couple of researchers asking if I wanted to participate in a clinical trial—clinical trial? Let me digest what just happened to me first.

I was also visited by the dietician, who, due to my suppressed immune system, gave me instructions on how to avoid infection. She advised me to stay clear of raw or undercooked foods like sushi or unpasteurized milk or cheese and to be sure to thoroughly wash my fruits and vegetables before eating them. I was also advised to avoid salad bars and smorgasbords or places where bacteria and germs are prevalent. Because infections are the number one cause of readmission after transplant, good hygiene, staying up to date on recommended immunizations, and distancing myself from people who exhibit flu or cold-like symptoms should be practiced for the rest of my life.

I was discharged from the hospital on Monday afternoon, May 8, 2023. But before being discharged, my brother collected all the prescriptions I needed going forward from the Hopkin's pharmacy. I remember the social worker advising (more like warning) me during my wait-list assessment process about all the drugs I would need to take for the rest of my life. I believe she mentioned maybe twenty or more pills a day. I don't know if that number was quoted to intimidate or garner how dedicated I was to the transplant process or what—but I was and am dedicated to adhering to the medication regimen, for sure.

The reality for me was three antirejection medications that must be taken in the morning and evening for the rest of my life, in addition to two anti-infection medicines that were prescribed for the first three to five months after surgery. Any additional medications required are specific to the patient's prior or current medical conditions (e.g., hypertension, diabetes, cholesterol meds, etc.). According to consumer reports, over half of American adults take four prescription medications on average per day, and that number increases with age. So maybe when the kidney patient hears this exorbitant number of pills needed posttransplant, it includes prescriptions they've already been taking.

I was sent home with a pill box filled with a week of prescriptions with instructions on how and when to take them. I also was instructed on how to empty my JP drains. There were two drains—drain 1 and drain 2. The tubes attached at the end of each drain were bulblike suction cups that hold a maximum of 50 cc(s) of drainage. I was required to log the drainage amount from each tube as well as the color and consistency of each. The drains would need to be emptied three or four times a day early on but decreased in volume, thickness, and darkness of color each day.

Each morning, I had to log my blood pressure, heart rate, temperature, and weight—each night, I needed to log my blood pressure and heart rate. This was to ensure that our new kidney was operating properly. The nurse needed to be notified if my systolic reading (top number) was greater than 150 or less than 100 and my diastolic reading (bottom number) was greater than 100 or less than 60. My heart rate should remain below 100 and above 55. If I gained more than three pounds in a day, that would indicate that I was retaining fluid and our kidney was not working. I was also keeping track of my blood glucose levels and was instructed to call my transplant nurse if my temperature exceeded 100 degrees.

Eight home health visits were scheduled by Johns Hopkins Home Care Group. The visits to my home began the day after I was discharged from the hospital. The skilled-nurse visits were twice a week that began on May 9 and ended on June 7. My home health nurse was a guy named Kassim. He was there to check my wounds, clean and change my bandages, and conduct an overall wellness check—my vital signs and logbook. I felt like I was getting presidential treatment!

Kassim was a Nigerian fellow in his mid-forties. He had a youthful appearance and a mellow, calm demeanor. In our thirty-minute visits, we discussed some of the cultural differences between his homeland and his experience here in the United States. He talked about one of the main differences was Americans seem to worry and talk about their health a lot more than the people in his native land. Not that there was no sickness, just that people didn't fret as much about it. He told me his grandmother lived to be 110 or 115, but his grandfather died long before that—hmm?

A physical therapist also came by on the third day of my first week home to test my mobility and make sure that I was capable of getting around my home comfortably. By this time, I was taking showers and getting fully dressed. I was doing well, so there was no reason for him to return.

After transplantation, the patient is required to have their blood tested on a regular basis to verify that there are no signs of organ rejection. Blood tests are the only way to truly know that your body is not rejecting the graft, so it is absolutely crucial that the patient follows the schedule.

I was required to have my blood tested twice a week for the first two months post-surgery, once a week for months three and four, once every other week for the remainder of the first year, and once a month thereafter—I believe the frequency further decreases as time passes. I initially started on Tuesday and Thursday and then Thursdays. Due to my standing 8:00 a.m. Thursday morning appointment, the local LabCorp staff know me, and I know them well.

On Thursday, May 18 (two weeks after my surgery), my sister and I attended my first post-op appointment at Hopkins. My JP drain was scheduled to be removed. I was really looking forward to this procedure—no anesthesia, no nothing, just pulling the two tubes out of my abdomen one at a time by my post-op transplant nurse. The pharmacists were there as well to explain, discuss, and calibrate my drug doses. My sister was in seventh heaven discussing pharmaceuticals with her peers. Most of it flew over my head at the time, but in a few weeks, I learned the jargon—at least the part relating to my prescriptions.

I began driving during the second week after my surgery and became very mobile once my tubes were removed, and shortly after that on June 1, my twenty-seven staples were removed, which really allowed me to feel more like my pre-prognosis self. Although it is recommended that the patient refrain from driving the first four to six weeks, I'm pretty sure some of the wait time is related to the patient's use of narcotic painkillers.

I resumed my morning walks and was accompanied by my buddy before he returned to Los Angeles on June 6. All my caregivers had returned home. I was all alone in this big empty house, and I was ready to start another beginning. It reminded me of the feeling one has a day or two after a funeral, the concern, attention, and activity leading up to the event and then suddenly, silence—you're all alone to face your new reality.

The urine from our donated kidney flows through the ureter into my bladder. During the transplant surgery, a stent was placed inside to prevent blockages from forming during the healing process. On June 8, six weeks after the operation, the stent was removed during an outpatient procedure using local anesthesia. A small scope was inserted into my urethra (via my male organ) to remove the stent. This took only a few moments, and I was able to drive myself to and from this appointment. I had the first of my quarterly post-op clinical visits on June 28. Things were progressing well, and I was released to resume normal activity. I was back on track—Hip, hip, hooray!

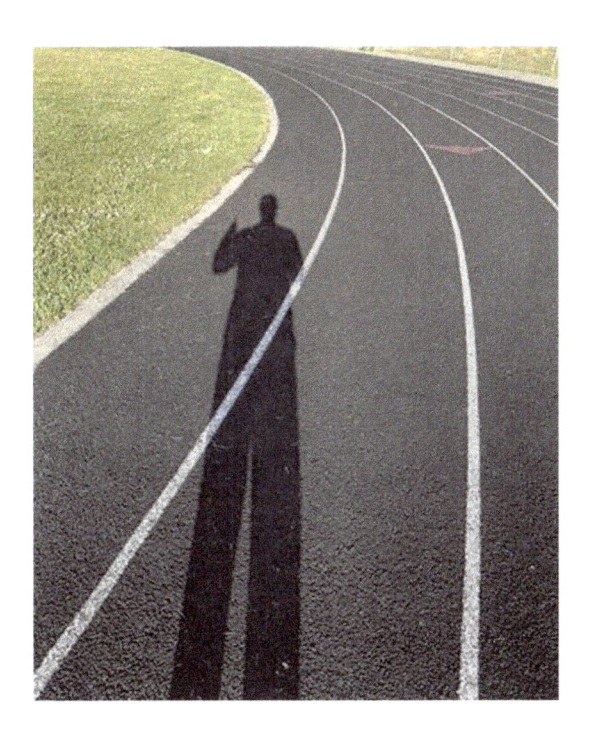

I am so grateful that I received this gift of life. I won't call it a second chance because I can't readily recall all the disastrous near misses I was spared throughout my life. There also have been so many fortunate events (known and unknown) that I've benefited from—only heaven knows. But I do know about this one, and I'll never forget it all the remaining days of my life.

I spent a large part of my career as an insurance underwriter; an underwriter in essence is someone who accepts or rejects risk. In other words, a good underwriter is someone who not only accepts beneficial risks but just as importantly avoids detrimental ones. I believe the same is true with a healthy lifestyle; what you put in your body is important, but what you don't put in your body is just as important. It's a risk/reward proposition.

I am the benefactor of traditional Western medicine. Once I was diagnosed and the treatment began, my life was extended until my son's lifesaving donation. Board-certified surgeons performed my operation. The pharmaceuticals prescribed by them and my compliance with their medical advice have saved my life. I am on the road to recovery and am feeling stronger with each passing month.

However, there are alternative methods to health care and preservation. They are practiced all over the world and have been practiced throughout the history of time. For example, Ayurveda and traditional Chinese medicine (TCM) are two of the more well-known examples.

Ayurveda is an ancient system of medicine that originated in India and is based on the concept of balance among the body, mind, spirit, and environment. Ayurveda uses various therapies, such as herbal medicines, special diets, meditation, yoga, massage, and more, to promote health and prevent disease.

In TCM, emotions and physical health are intimately connected. This integrated mind-body approach to health and healing operates in a dynamic loop where emotions impact the health of the body and vice versa. As we know, the kidneys remove toxins and excess fluid via urine. In TCM, the kidney is related to fear, which can manifest as chronic fear or anxiety when qi (pronounced *Chee* in English) is out of balance.

Both Ayurveda and TCM are considered alternative medicine in the Western world, and their effectiveness and safety have not been well studied by scientific standards. Then there are those who swear by the benefits of naturopathic and homeopathic medicine. I'm not intimately familiar with any of these methods of health care, so I can't personally endorse them. But there has been a movement in recent years to intertwine traditional Western medicine and those practiced in non-Western or Eastern cultures.

What I do know from personal experience is if you want a fighting chance at good health, you must drink an adequate amount of water every day, carefully consider what you put in your mouth/bloodstream, move your body, and get regular periodic medical checkups. In addition, for me and those of us who have received donated organs, we must avoid nonsteroidal anti-inflammatory drugs (NSAIDs) and continue the recommended daily dosage of immunosuppressant drugs to prevent our bodies' antibodies from attacking the donated organ.

My dialysis treatments sustained me until I was able to receive my son's donated kidney. My health has improved tremendously and continues to improve. It's like replacing a broken part with a new one (or in my case adding one)—everything begins to function better.

My energy returned with the increased production of red blood cells and the elimination of toxins. My blood pressure has normalized with improved kidney function. My appetite has returned, and I am beginning to regain my weight. I am exercising again and have reentered life with a renewed purpose.

This bears repeating. *To this day, I don't know if my son truly understands what he did for me.*

CHAPTER 12

Better to Give than to Receive

I knew the day that my son and I were approved for the surgery that if I survived, I was going to do whatever I could to help dialysis patients and the broader kidney disease community. I remember saying to anyone who would listen that I am willing to do anything from mopping floors to public speaking—however I can help, just let me know. Put me in, coach!

After all the grace and goodwill shown to me during my ordeal and continues to be shown, I would be remiss if I didn't pay it forward. I want and I will give with no expectation of receiving anything in return, other than the inner joy I feel from helping someone in need. When I would see some of my fellow dialysis patients who were blind due to complications from diabetes or with amputated limbs as a result of peripheral vascular disease or neuropathy or those with twisted and disfigurement limbs due to strokes or the funeral service notices of former patients tacked to the bulletin board that hung above the scale, I truly believe that I was spared to serve others.

In the past, I've contributed to various causes or charities but not in the way I will give to this cause. Some of my giving in the past was obligatory or reluctant or even with the expectation of receiving something in return. Giving is giving, and I'm sure most recipients are pleased no matter the giver's motivation. But I tend to believe what the scriptures teach us about the best way to give in 2 Corinthians 9:7: "Each of you should give what you have decided in your heart to give, not reluctantly or under compulsion, for God loves a cheerful giver."

I know there are many of us who believe that happiness comes from receiving what we want, whether it's money, fame, power, or love—but like our parents taught us, it's better to give than to receive. I bet if you ask the average person what they received for Christmas or a birthday two years ago, they might not remember, but ask that same person what they gave someone from the heart ten years ago, they'll remember with a smile on their face.

I believe that when we give to others, we feel good about ourselves and our actions, and we also experience a warm glow of altruism. It helps us appreciate what we have and what others need. When we give, we become more aware of the value of our resources and the impact of our generosity on others. We also become more empathetic and compassionate as we try to understand the feelings and perspectives of those we help. Giving is infectious, creating a cycle of kindness and generosity.

People often say, "Everything happens for a reason." I agree, but I also believe that *that* reason most often is the intentional or unintentional actions of one person or group. I first heard about Someday Isle in Brian Tracy's 2016 book, *Get Smart*. In my own words, the most densely populated place on earth is Someday Isle: someday I'll change, someday I'll have time, someday I'll be this or do that, someday, someday, someday!

I remember visiting my parents' house many years ago, and my father had attached the following to the refrigerator door:

> This is a story about four people named Everybody, Somebody, Anybody, and Nobody. There was an important job to be done and Everybody was sure that Somebody would do it. Anybody could have done it, but Nobody did it. Somebody got angry about that because

it was Everybody's job. Everybody thought Anybody could do it, but Nobody realized that Everybody wouldn't do it. It ended up that Everybody blamed Somebody when Nobody did what Anybody could have. (Author unknown)

It's so easy to defer to others or to bury one's head in the proverbial sand, to ignore the obvious train coming down the track, or to cross that bridge when we get there—dull cliches, perhaps, but true, nonetheless. We are designed to help one another. There is a symbiotic necessity to the survival of us all: "Each one, teach one." "One hand washes the other, and both hands wash the face." The importance of a helpful hand, a watchful eye, a gentle touch, a listening ear, or even a kind word goes a long way in comforting those in need.

As implied in the gospel of Matthew, whosoever will be chief among you, will be chief in service. Dr. Martin Luther King Jr. so eloquently expressed it in his "Drum Major Instinct" sermon: "Everybody can be great, because everybody can serve." You don't have to have worldwide notoriety or a large platform to serve. Is it true the more people you reach, the greater the potential impact? Absolutely! But speaking from personal experience, the care and kindness shown by one individual to another mean the world to that individual.

What comes to my mind at this moment is that haunting American Cancer Society public service announcement by the late actor Yul Brynner—it aired approximately two months after he died from lung cancer. During his heyday, he reportedly smoked five packs of cigarettes a day. This commercial appeared on television in January or February of 1986. In his distinctive baritone voice, he simply said the following: "Now that I'm gone, I tell you, don't smoke. Whatever you do, just don't smoke."

I echo this sentiment with the following additions: don't ignore your blood pressure or your blood test results—your body is trying to tell you something!

Please listen.

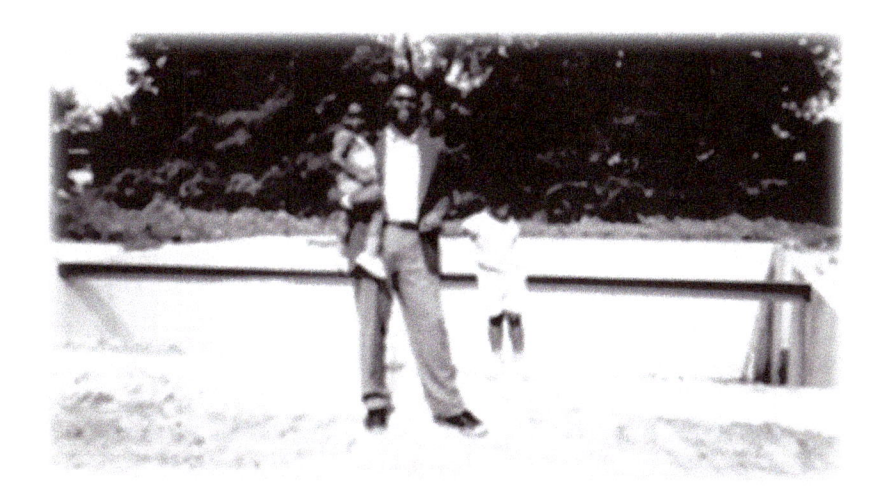

"I hear babies cry, I watch the grow, they'll learn much more than I'll ever know, and I think to myself, What a Wonderful World."

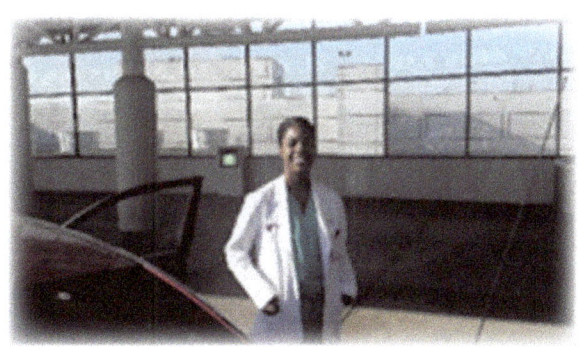

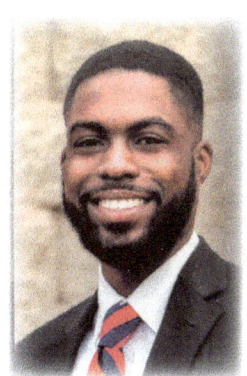

The Life Saver			The Promise

QUICK KIDNEY DISEASE FACTS AND STATS

(https://www.kidneyfund.org/all-about-kidneys/
quick-kidney-disease-facts-and-stats)

Check out the following basic facts and statistics about chronic kidney disease:

1. Thirty-seven million Americans have kidney disease, and millions more are at risk.
2. About 808,000 Americans are living with kidney failure.
3. More than 556,000 Americans are on dialysis.
4. More than 250,000 Americans are living with a kidney transplant.
5. Kidney disease is growing at an alarming rate. It currently affects more than one in seven of American adults, with people of color at greater risk for kidney failure.
6. Nine out of ten people with kidney disease are unaware they have it, and half of those with severely reduced kidney function (but not yet on dialysis) do not know they have kidney disease.
7. About one in three adults with diabetes may have kidney disease. Diabetes is the top cause of kidney failure, causing nearly half (45%) of new cases.
8. One in five adults with high blood pressure may have kidney disease. High blood pressure is the second most common cause of kidney failure, causing 28% of new cases.
9. For every two women who develop kidney failure, three men develop kidney failure. However, kidney

disease is more common in women than men (14.3% vs. 12.4%).
10. Kidney disease is the fastest-growing noncommunicable disease in the United States.
11. Kidney disease is a silent killer, usually with no signs or symptoms until the late stages.
12. Kidney disease is one of the top ten causes of death in the United States. It kills more people each year than breast or prostate cancer.
13. Kidney disease can lead to heart attack, stroke, kidney failure, and death.
14. While early kidney disease has no signs or symptoms, simple blood and urine tests can tell how well your kidneys are working. If you're at risk, talk to your doctor about getting tested.
15. Early detection saves lives. Kidney disease is not reversible, but it is treatable. When caught and treated early, it's often possible to slow or stop the progression of kidney disease and avoid serious complications like heart attack, stroke, kidney failure, and death.
16. Your kidneys are vital organs—just like your heart, lungs, and liver. Your kidneys clean your blood, help control your blood pressure, help make red blood cells, and keep your bones healthy.
17. Being physically active, keeping a healthy weight, consuming kidney-friendly foods and fluids, and getting tested for kidney disease can help protect your kidneys. Even small changes can make a big difference.
18. Compared to white Americans:
    - Black Americans are more than four times more likely to develop kidney failure.
    - Native Americans are about twice as likely to develop kidney failure.

ABOUT THE AUTHOR

El Jai Macoy is a former college athlete and retired insurance professional. He is a volunteer for the National Kidney Foundation, the American Kidney Fund, and Infinite Legacy. Over thirty-seven million US residents suffer from chronic kidney disease, and another nine out of ten are unaware they even have it. This debut novel discusses his personal journey with kidney disease in hopes of providing encouragement to those experiencing the same issue as well as providing guidance to those hoping to avoid this fate.

He is a proud father of two adult children and resides in the state of Maryland, USA.